HEALTHCARE HEROES
Coloring Book

Stress Relieving Designs, Quotes and Affirmations

Ronald Holt

William Huggett

Those in the healing professions often find their self-care takes a back seat due to the extraordinary demands being placed on them. This can lead to additional stress and burnout.

Healthcare Heroes Coloring Book: Stress Relieving Designs, Quotes and Affirmations includes 35 beautifully created designs with inspirational quotes and messages of affirmation. This book is designed to help healers find strength and encouragement during these challenging times.

Studies have shown that coloring mandalas can calm the brain and decrease stress. Meditative coloring is a great way to rejuvenate. This book also provides quick and easy suggestions for self-care.

Sincerely,

Ronald Holt, DO
William Huggett, MD

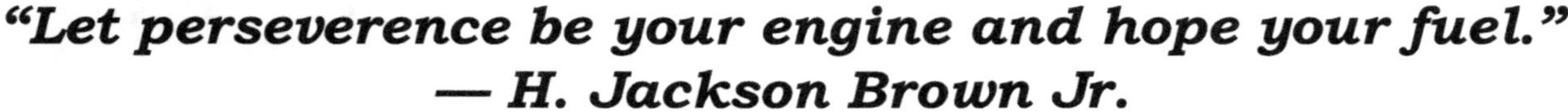

You may face many challenges, but your determination
and hope will help you persevere.

Your strength and desire to help others is everlasting.

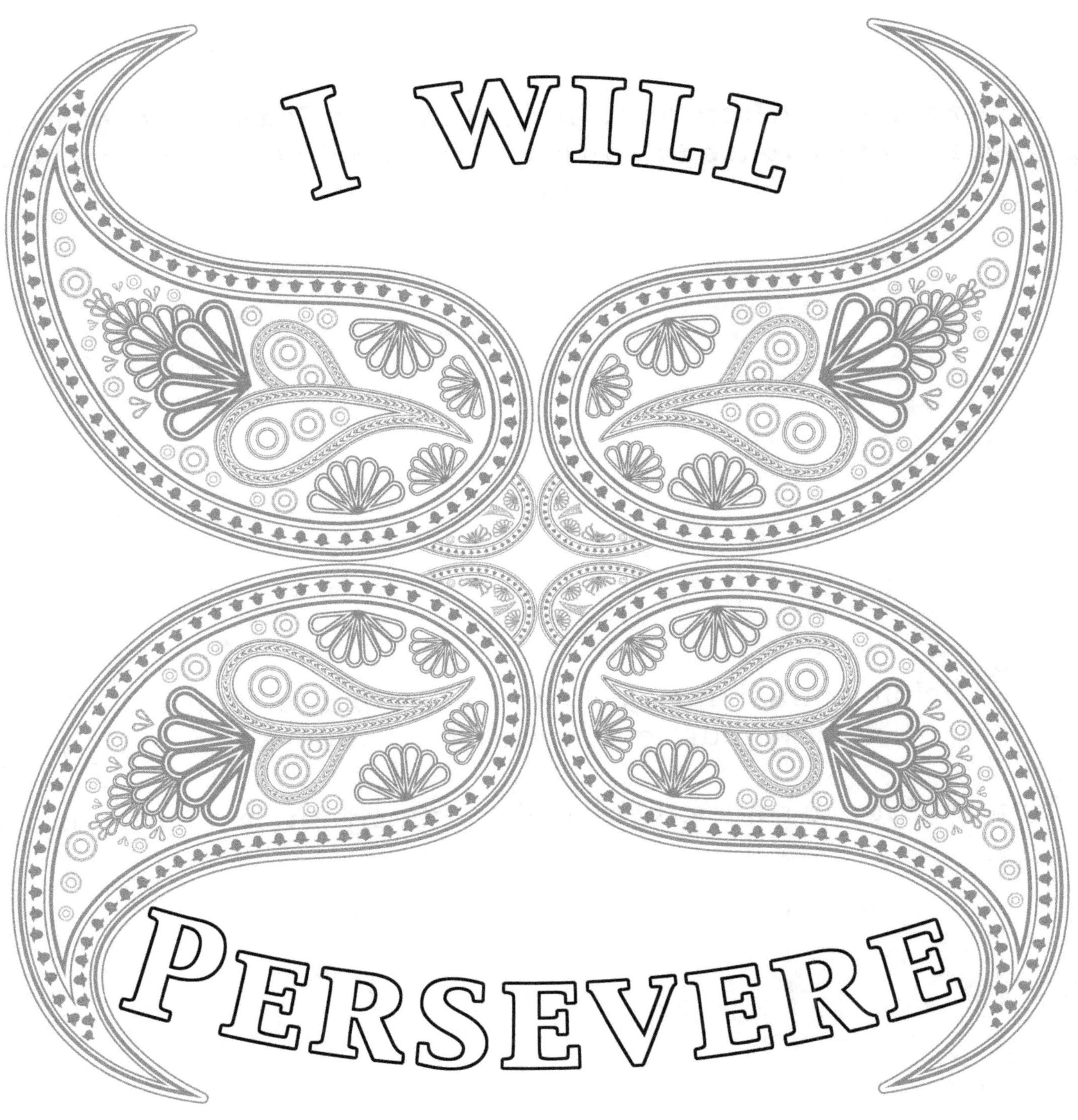

Affirmation: My dedication to helping others is never-ending.

"A hero is an ordinary individual who finds the strength to persevere and endure in spite of the overwhelming obstacles."
— Christopher Reeve

Helping others may feel like it's just part of your job,
but your actions are extraordinary.

You continue to serve others while putting your own life at risk.

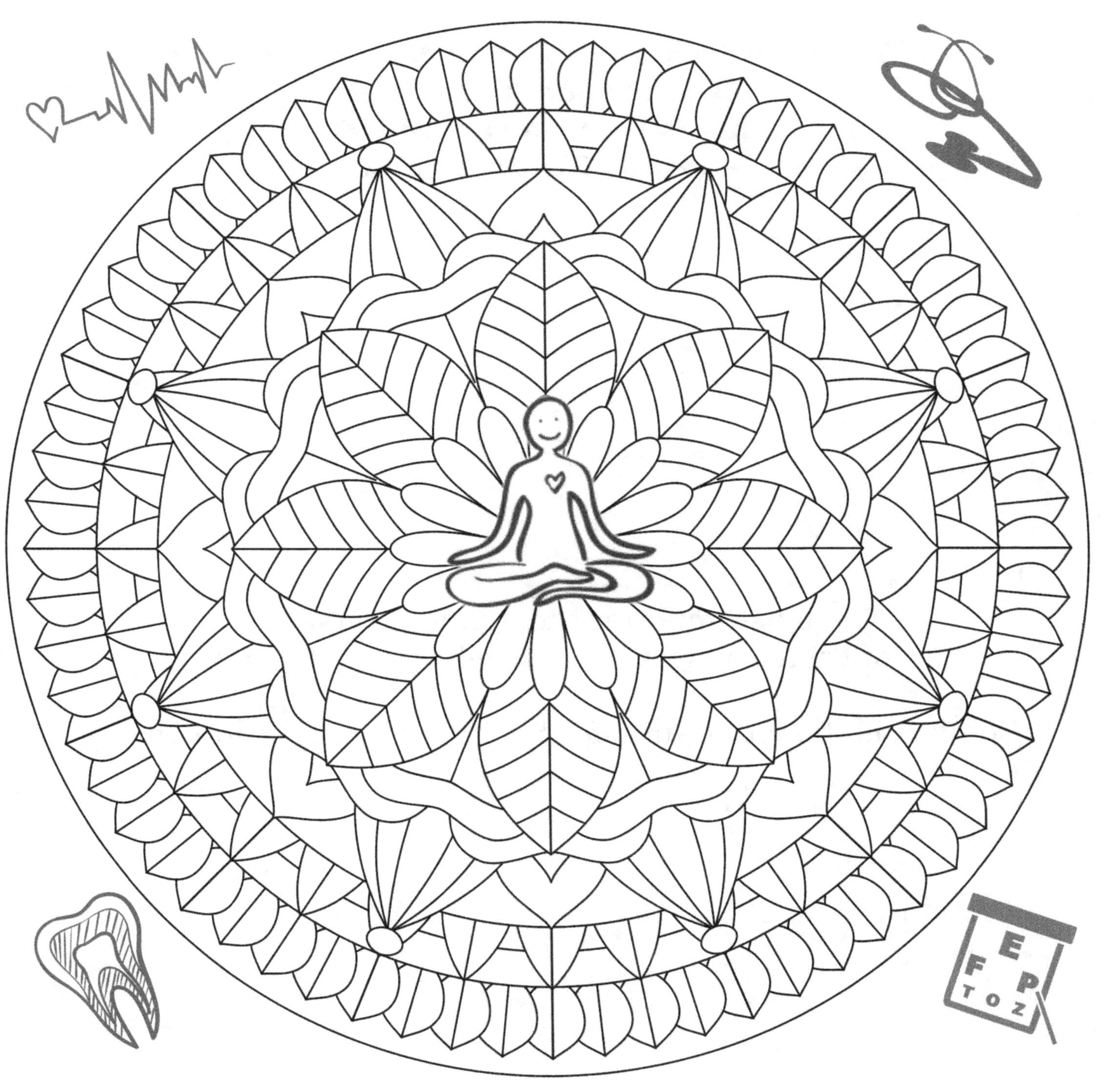

Affirmation: I am a healthcare hero.

*"To know even one life has breathed easier
because you have lived.
This is to have succeeded."
— Ralph Waldo Emerson*

The most important tool in your arsenal is
offering comfort to those who are suffering.

Comfort is the foundation for health, wellness, and healing.

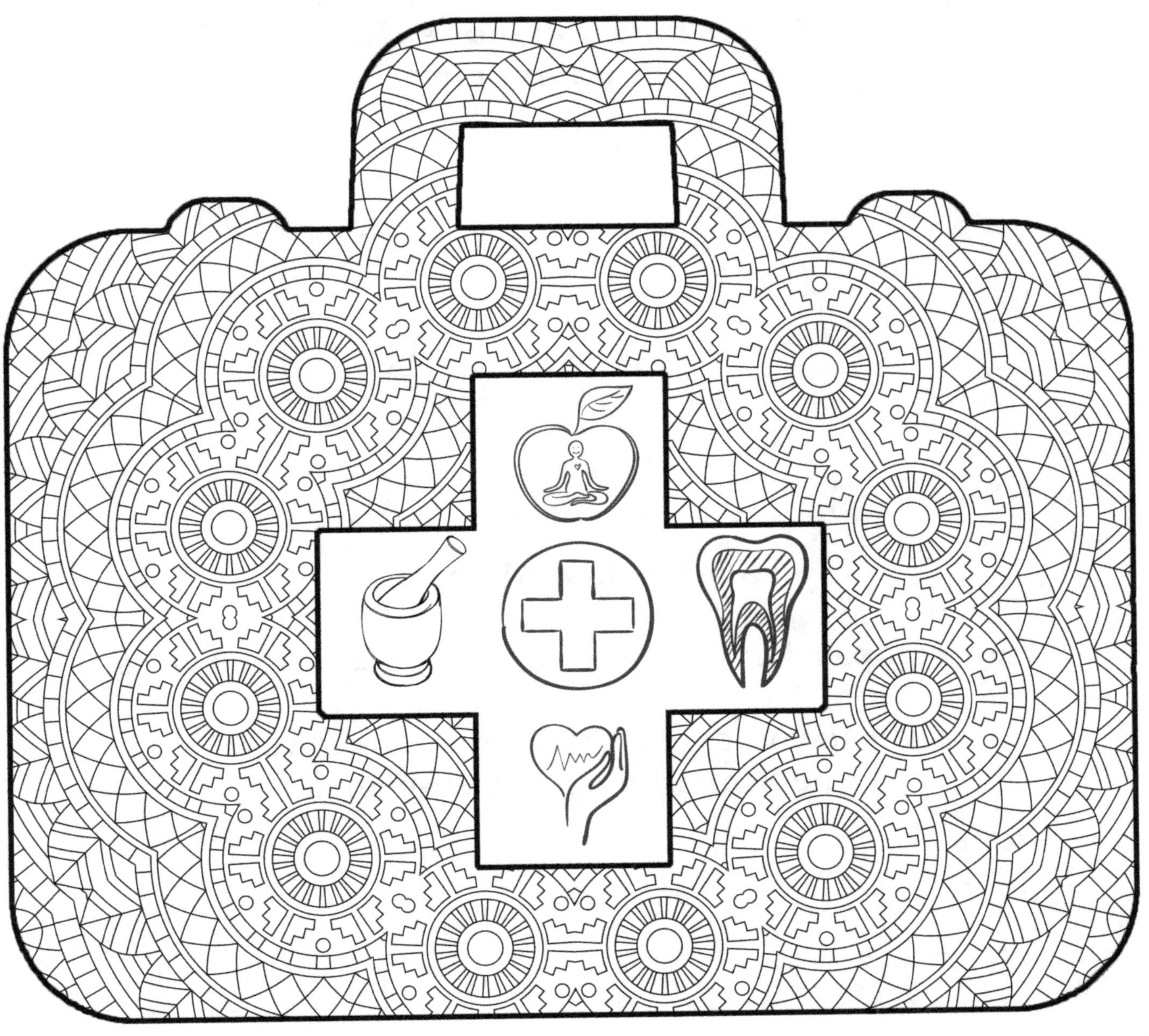

Affirmation: I succeed by helping others.

*"I've learned that people will forget what you said,
people will forget what you did, but people will
never forget how you made them feel."*
— Maya Angelou

Patients depend on you.

Your compassion is making a difference in their lives.

Those you care for will never forget your
dedication to their well-being.

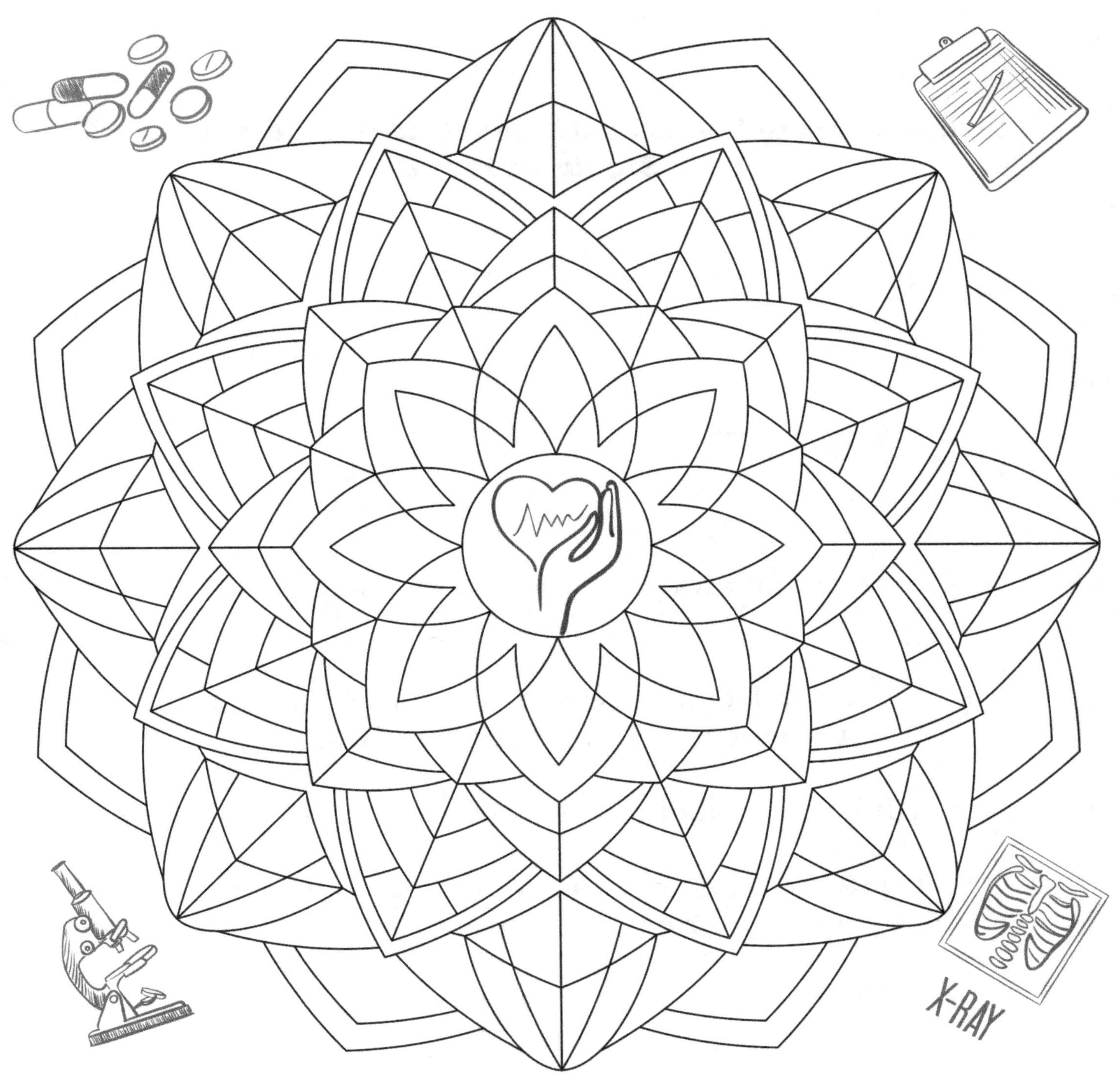

Affirmation: I bring comfort to my patients.

"Being entirely honest with onself is a good exercise."
— Sigmund Freud

You may not always feel at the top of your game.
And that's OK.

If you are feeling stressed and unable to cope,
it's perfectly OK to reach out for help.

Strength lies in reaching out rather than suffering alone.

There are many resources available to support
your emotional wellness.

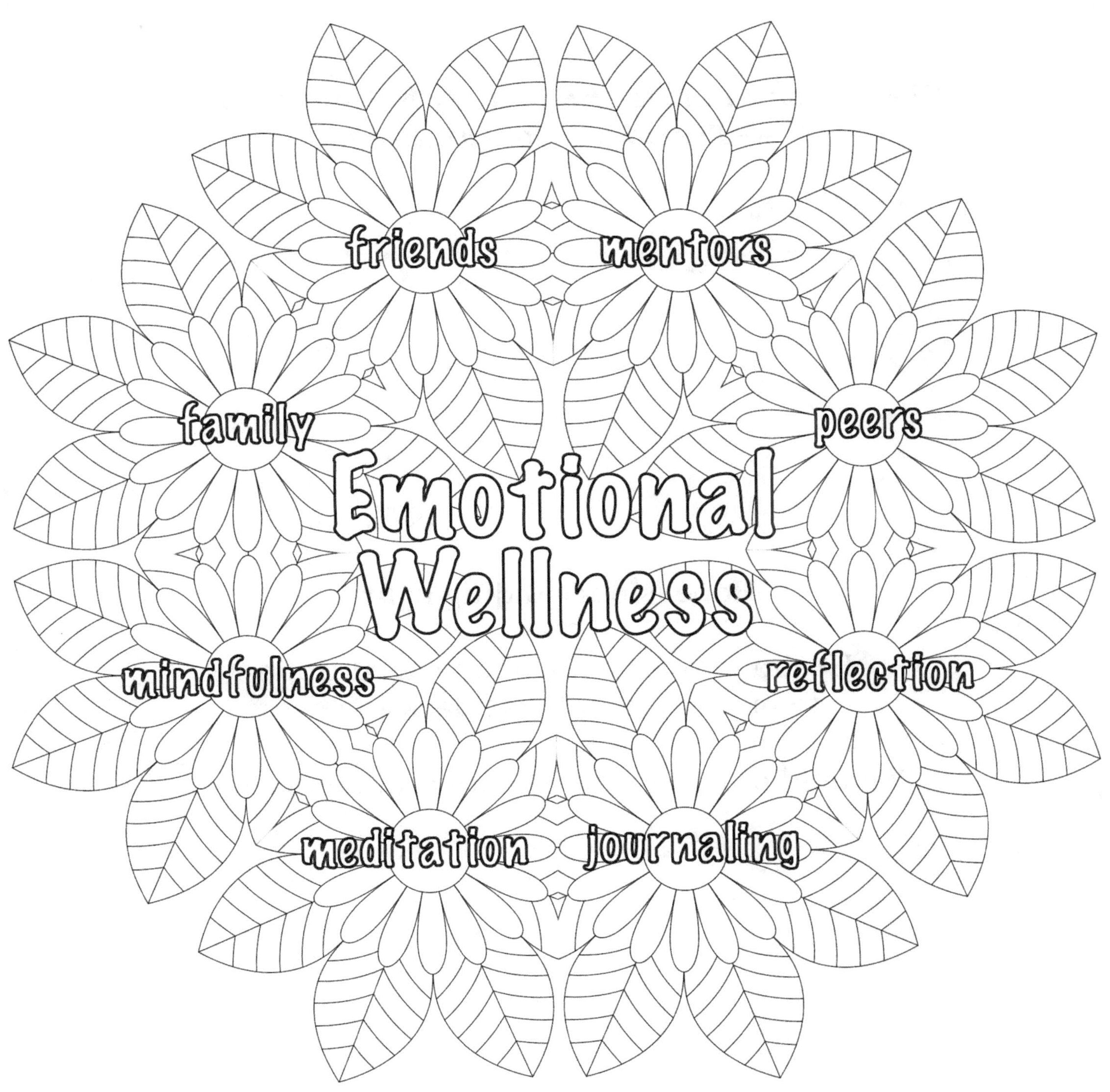

Affirmation: I am committed to my emotional wellness.

"Fear never builds the future, but hope does."
— President Joseph Biden

Hope is our guiding light.

Healing professionals are called upon
to offer hope in these dark times.

We hold onto hope for others and ourselves.

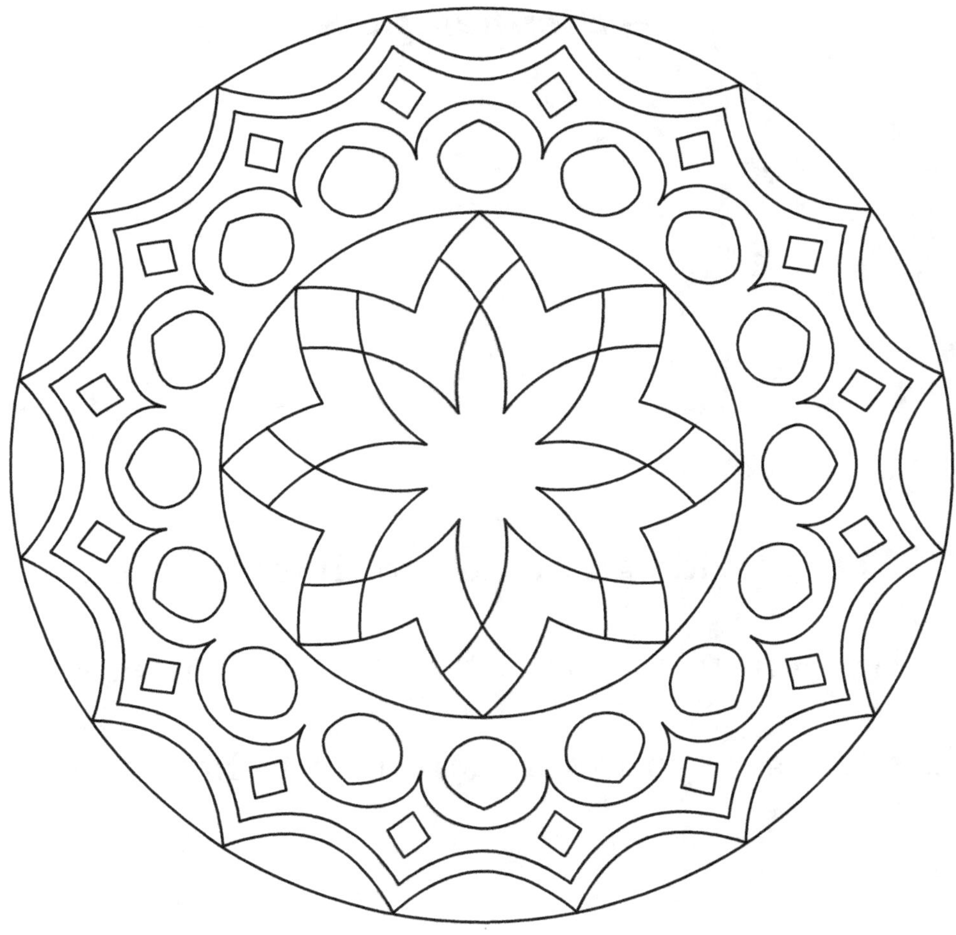

Affirmation: I offer hope to those in need.

You provide great care to those in need.

But you must also attend to your needs.

This will give you more strength to help others.

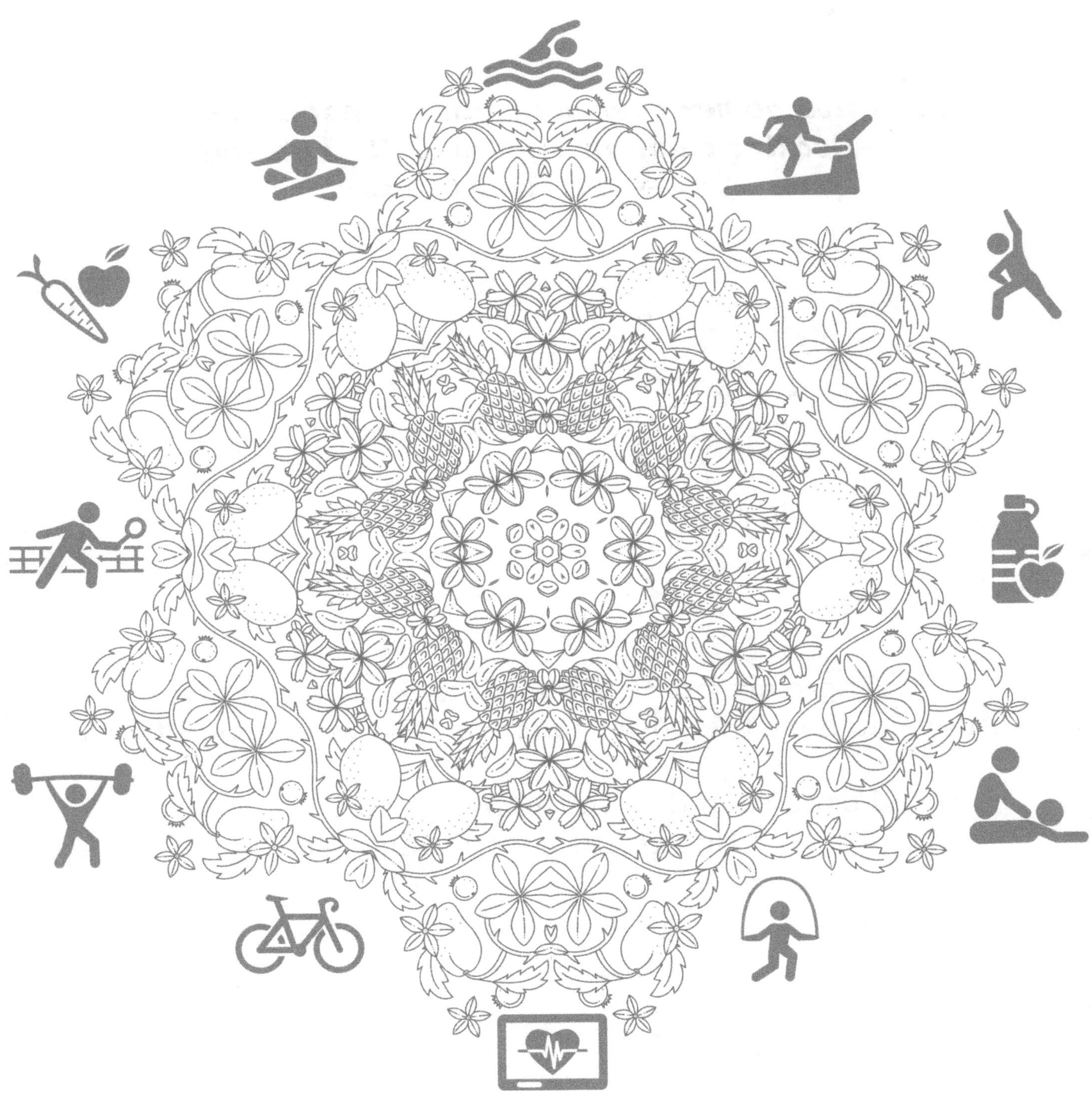

Affirmation: I utilize many ways to care for myself.

"You have power over your mind -- not outside events.
Realize this, and you will find strength.
— Marcus Aurelius

There are many things outside of our control,
but we do have the power to chose how we respond to events.

Focus each day on the things you can control
and release everything else.

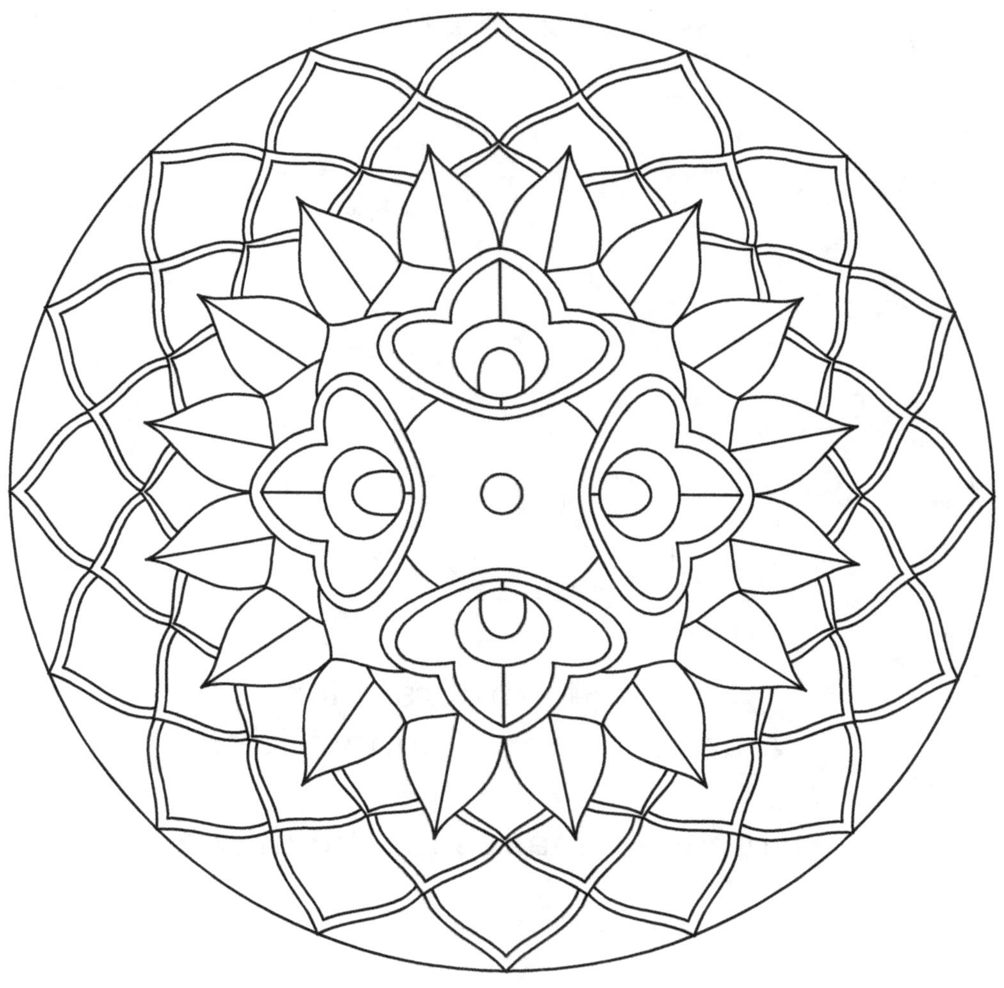

Affirmation: Choosing what I focus on brings me strength.

*"The best way to find yourself
is to lose yourself in the service of others."
— Mahatma Gandhi*

Service to others offers
a deeper connection within.

Your dedication makes all the difference.

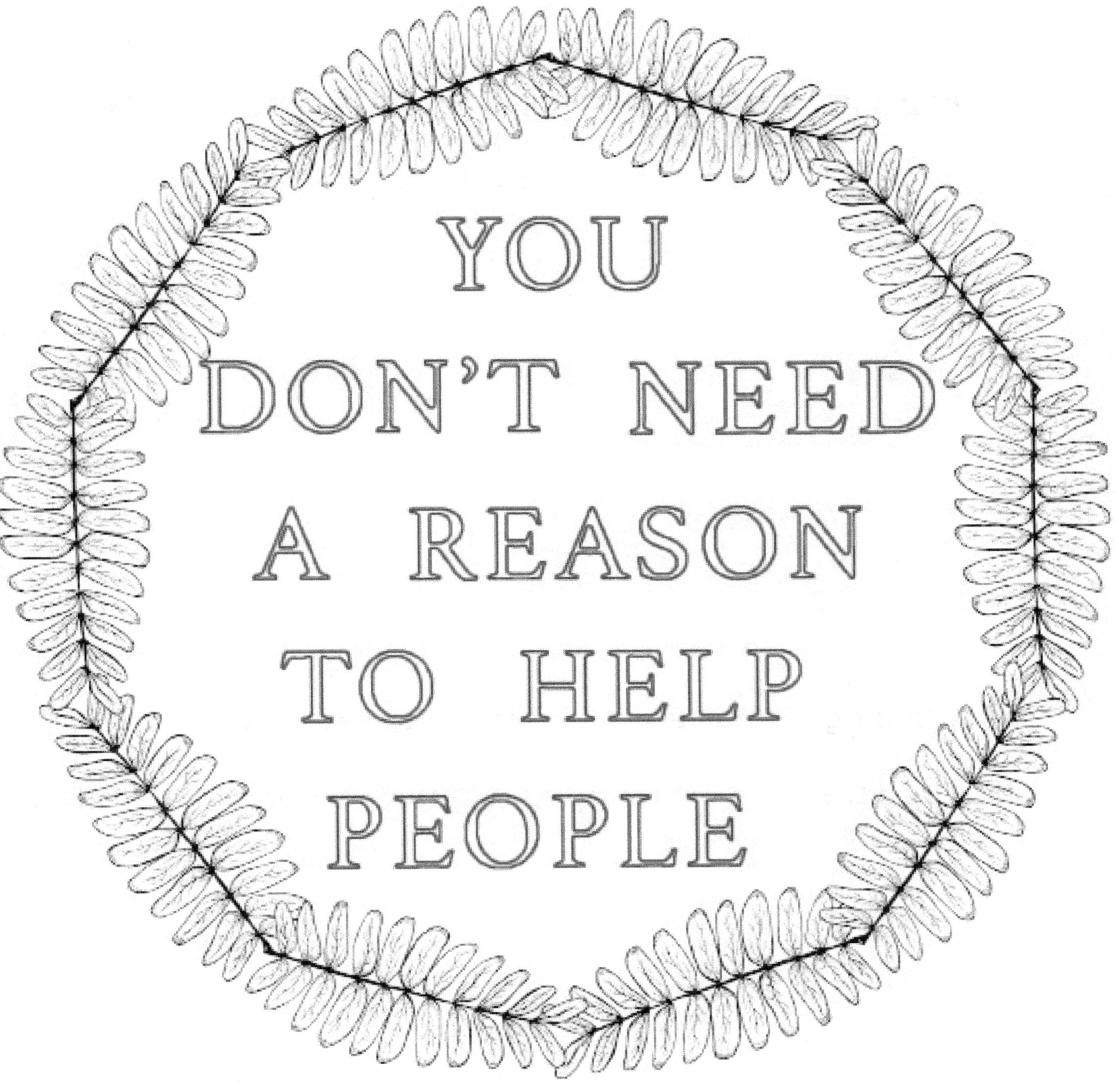

Affirmation: I am committed to community service.

*"The greatest glory in living lies not in never falling,
but in rising every time we fall."*
— Nelson Mandala

Your calling is to be a healer, but some days you will fall.

Those are the days to rise up as a better version of yourself.

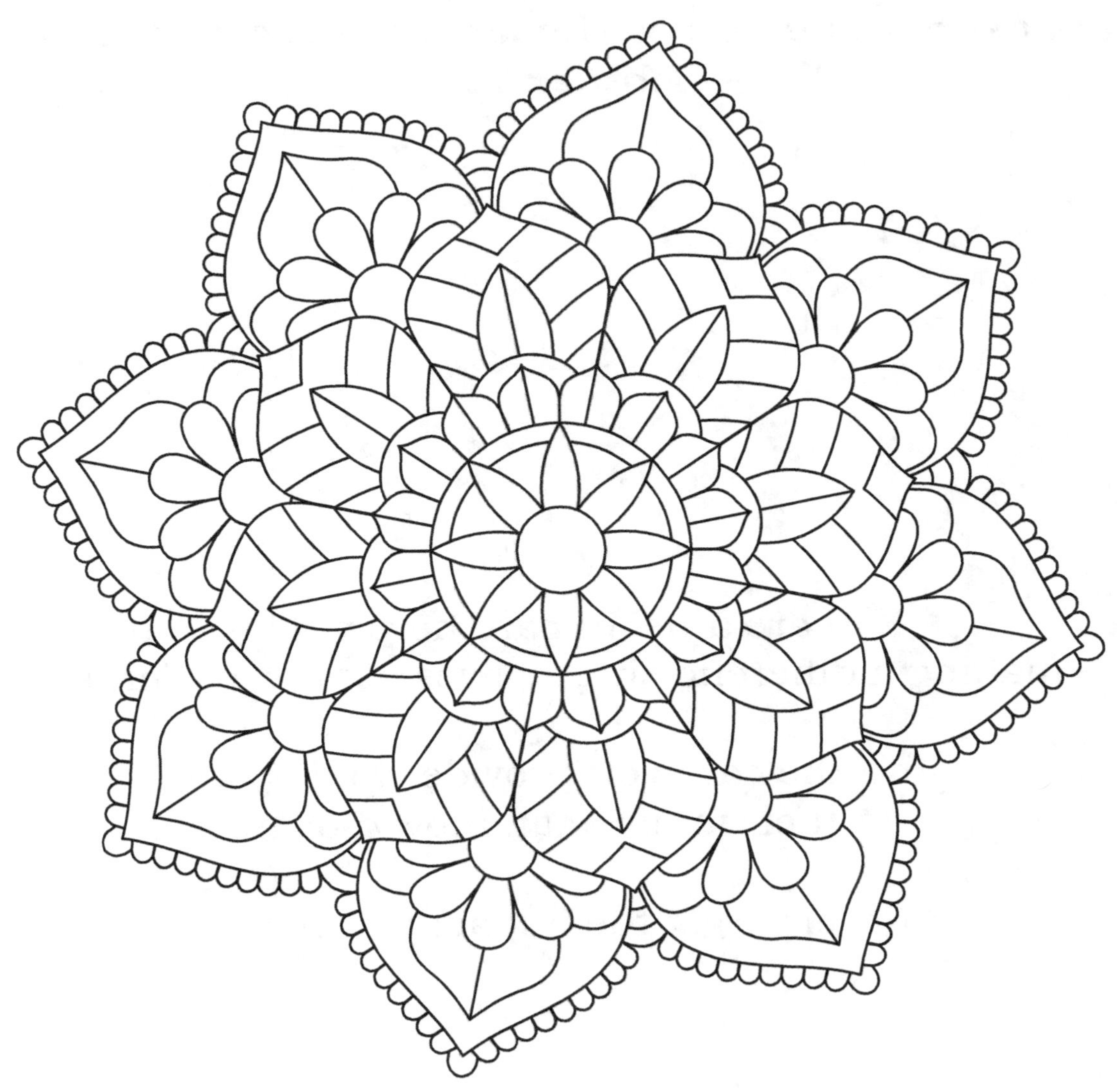

Affirmation: Nothing will keep me down.

*"I alone cannot change the world,
but I can cast a stone across the water to create many ripples."*
— Mother Teresa

You are a healthcare hero who is
making a difference in the lives of your patients.

And the care you provide ripples out
to their families and loved ones.

Never forget the impact you have.

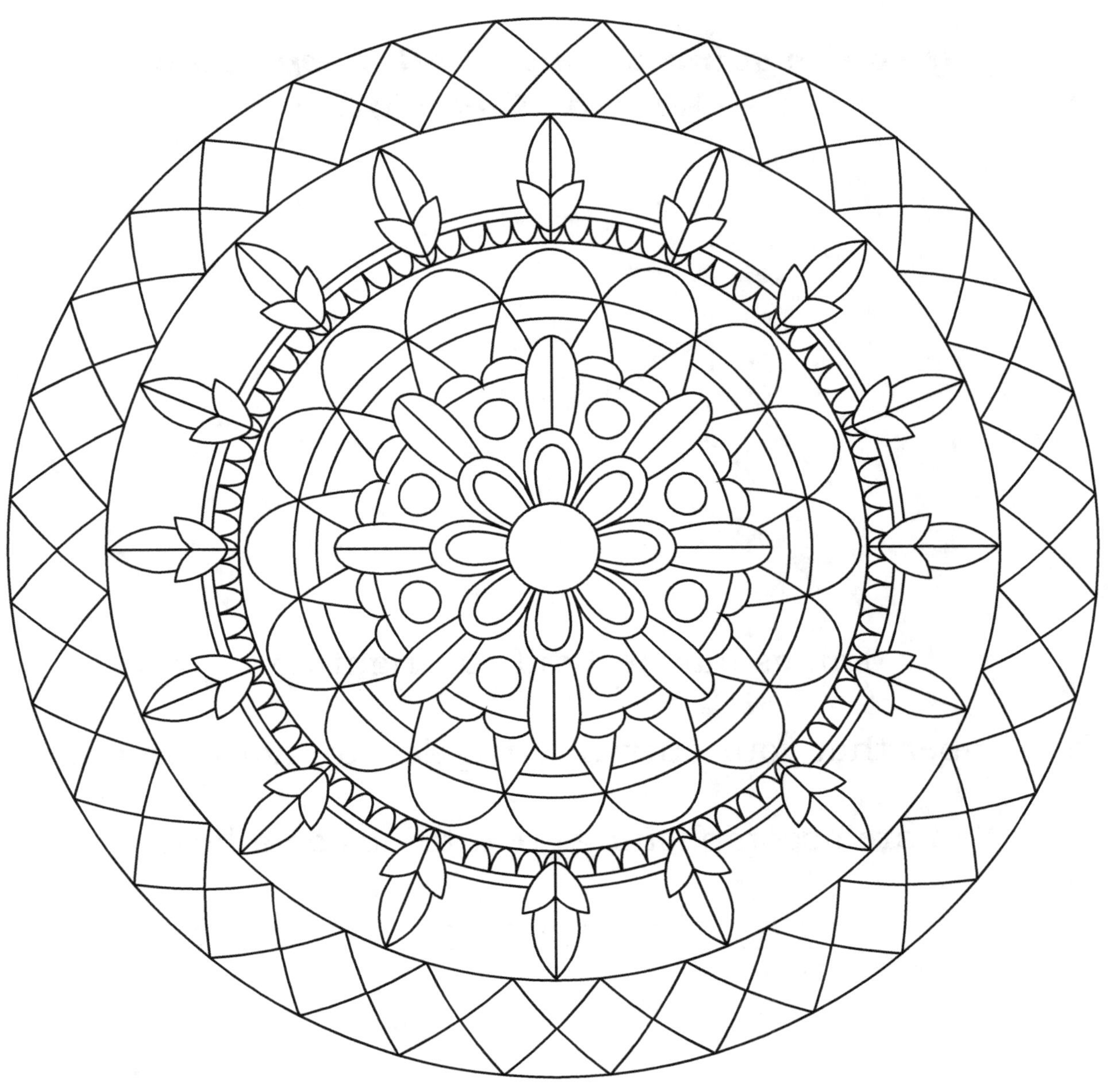

Affirmation: I impact many people.

"If you're going through hell, keep going."
— Winston Churchill

Things may feel difficult right now.

Remember that your current struggles are not permanent.

You are accomplishing great things as a healer.

Never give up.

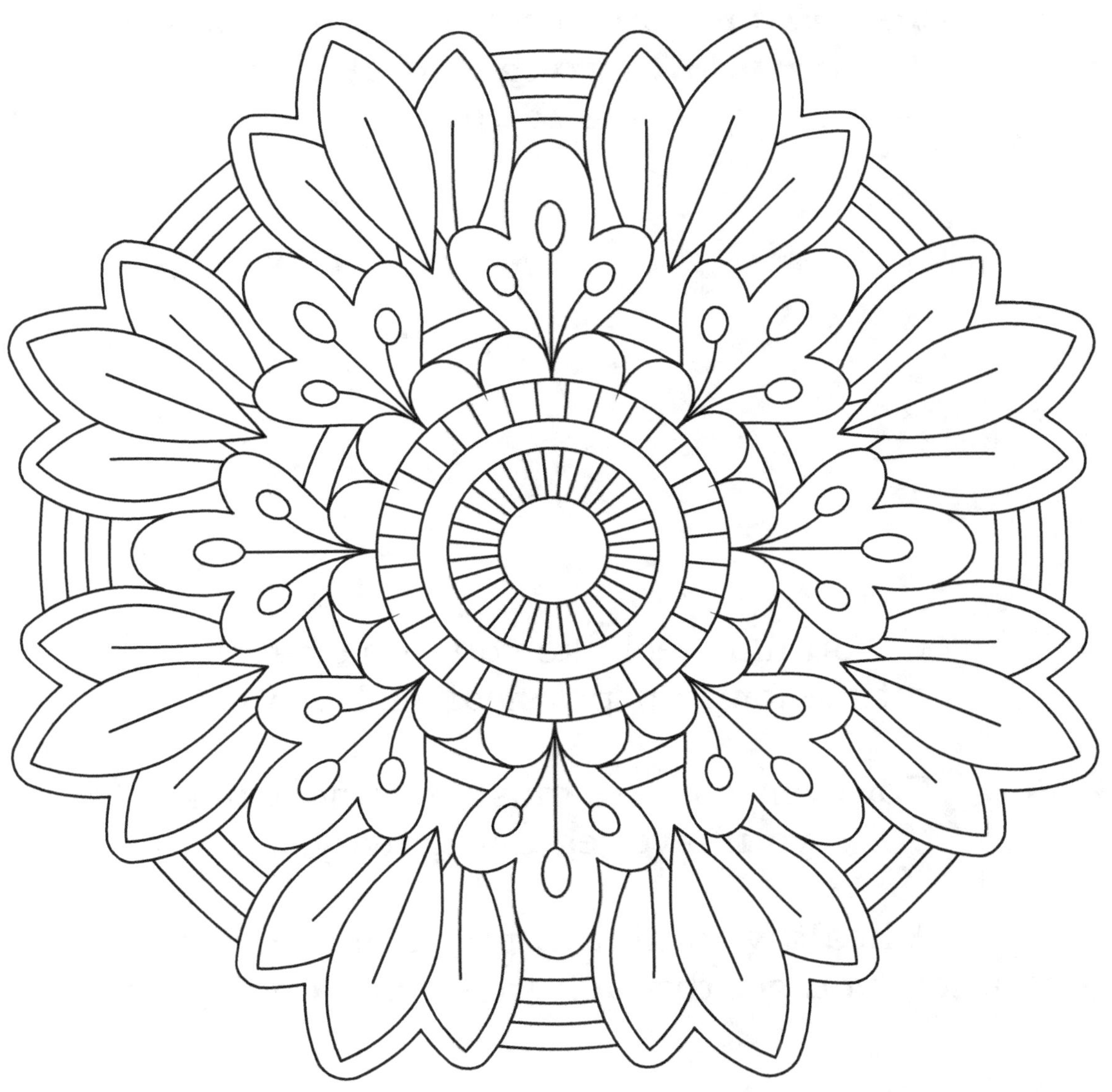

Affirmation: I will keep going.

You may feel like you don't have
time for your physical well-being.

However, you are most effective when
you have regular activity.

A healthy routine of physical exercise
can help you get through these challenging times.

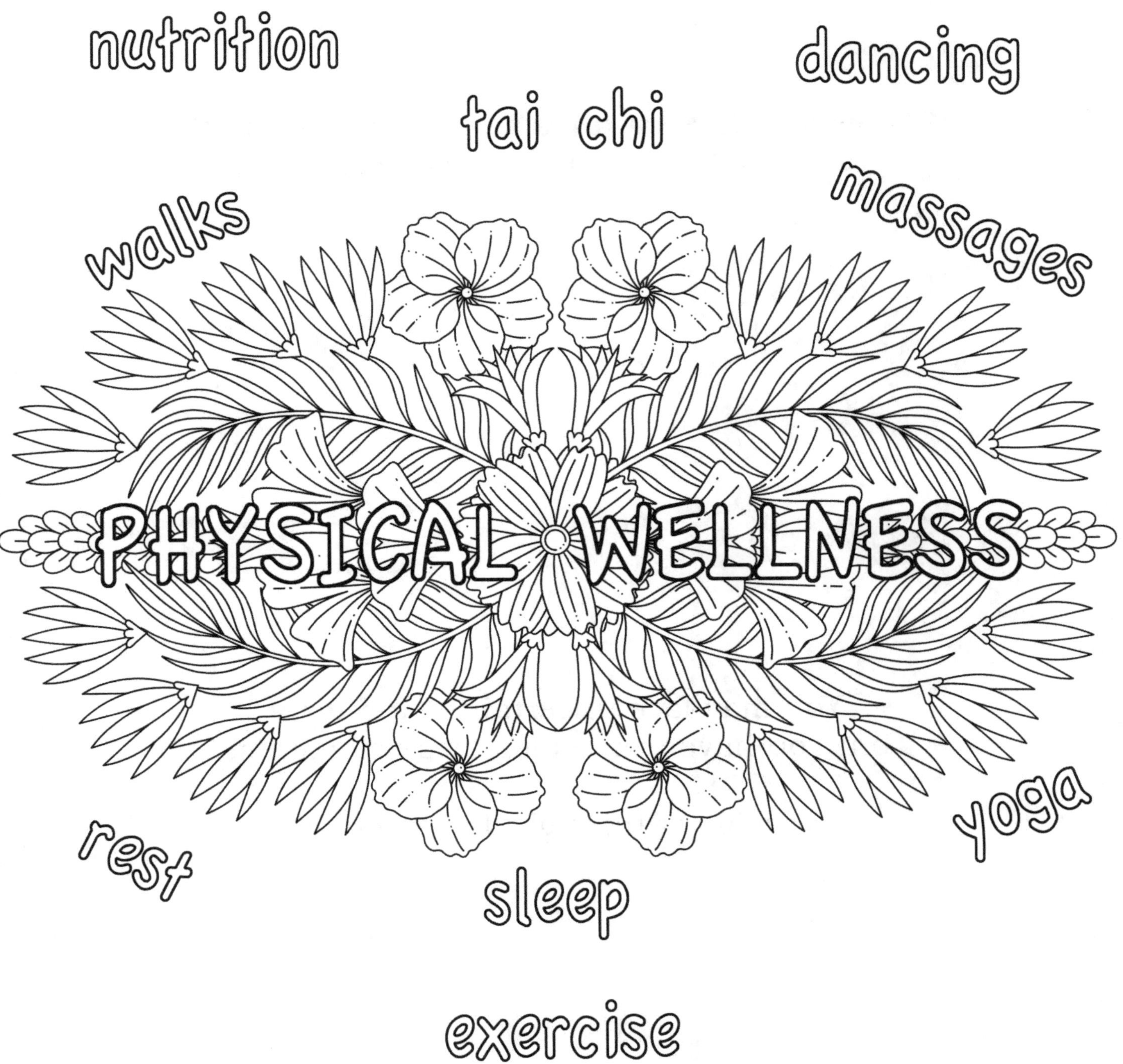

Affirmation: I am committed to my physical well-being.

"The only thing we have to fear is fear itself."
— Franklin D. Roosevelt

You may face uncertainty and fear,
but you have trained for these moments.

We will get through this together.

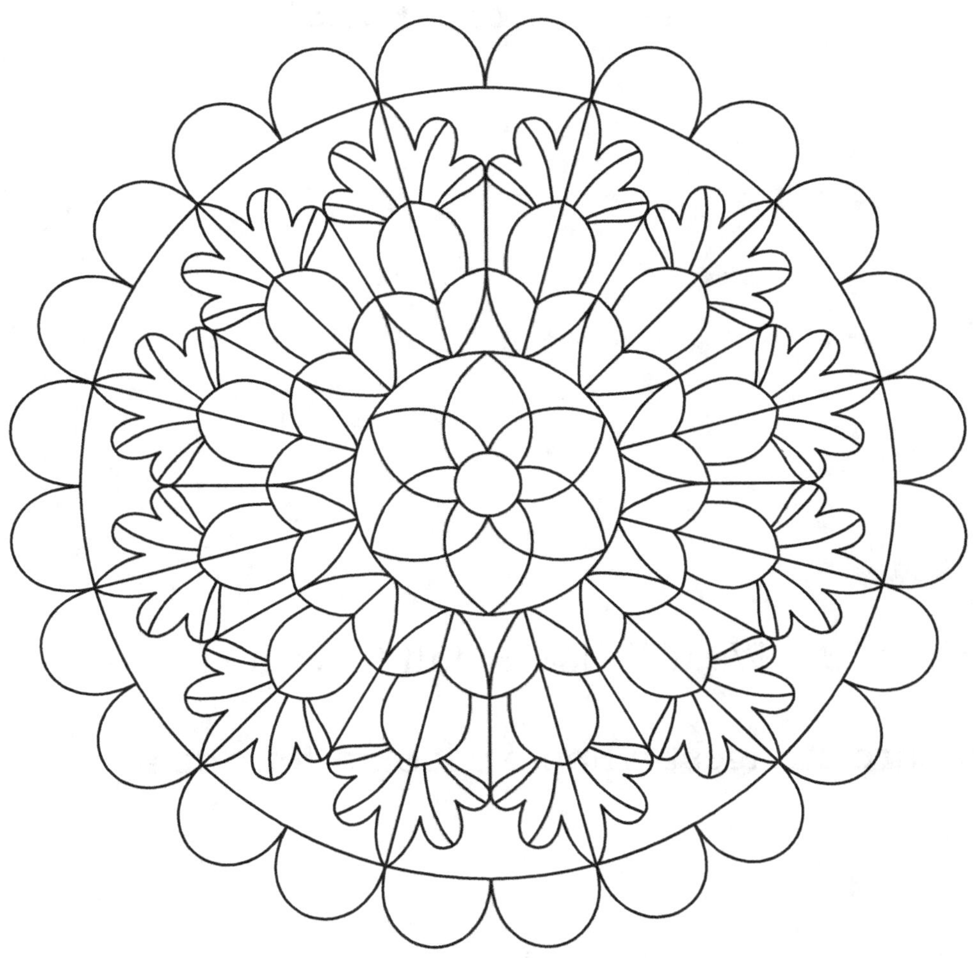

Affirmation: I harness my courage.

*"Now is the time, if ever there was one,
for us to care selflessly about one another."
— Anthony Fauci*

We will rise or fall together.

We are stongest when we look after one another.

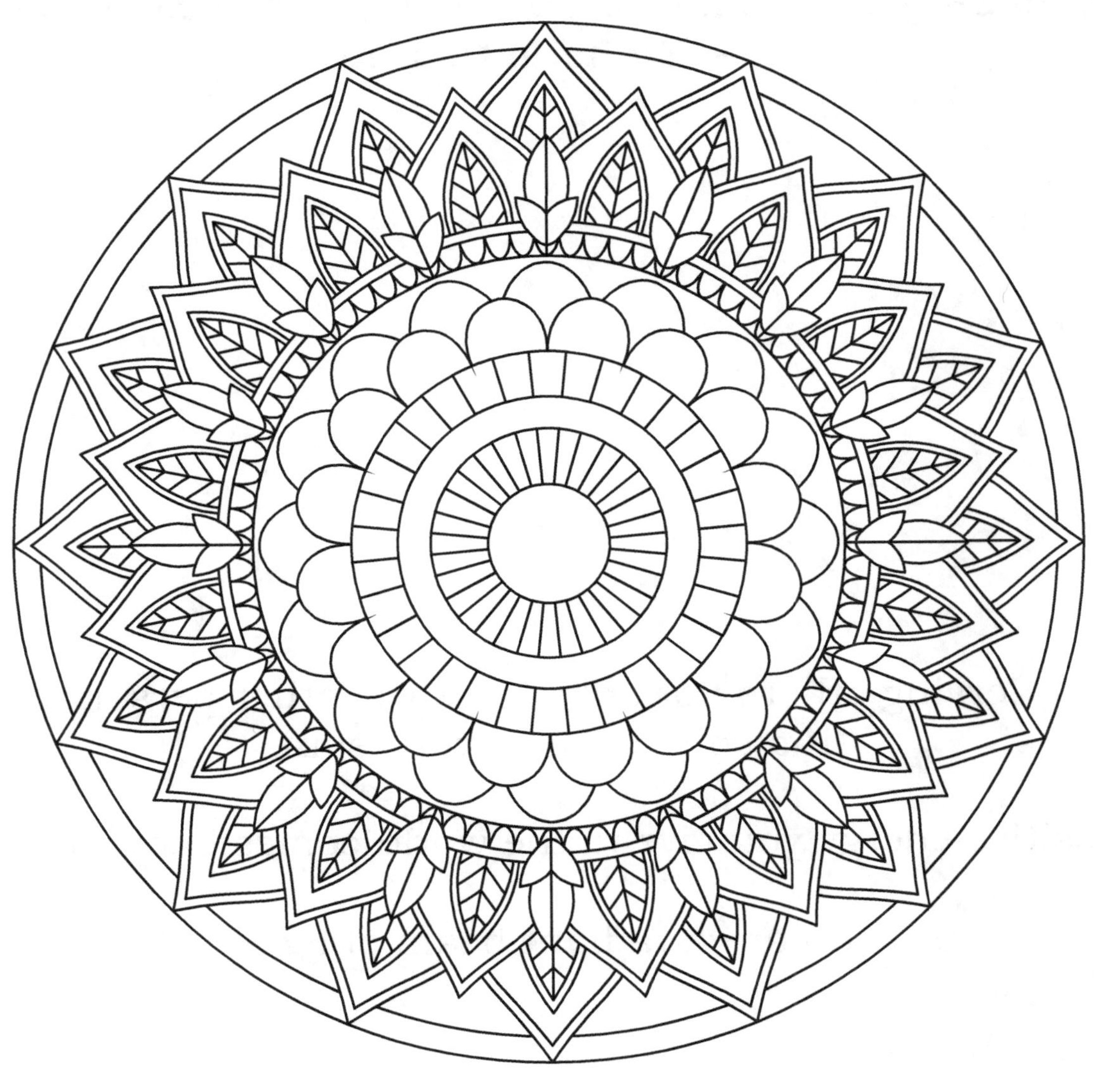

Affirmation: My commitment to caring for others is unrelenting.

"That energy that you give out, you get it back in return."
— Michelle Obama

Serving others not only helps the other person,
it also nourishes your soul.

The positive energy you give to the world comes back many fold.

You are a radiant beam of light.

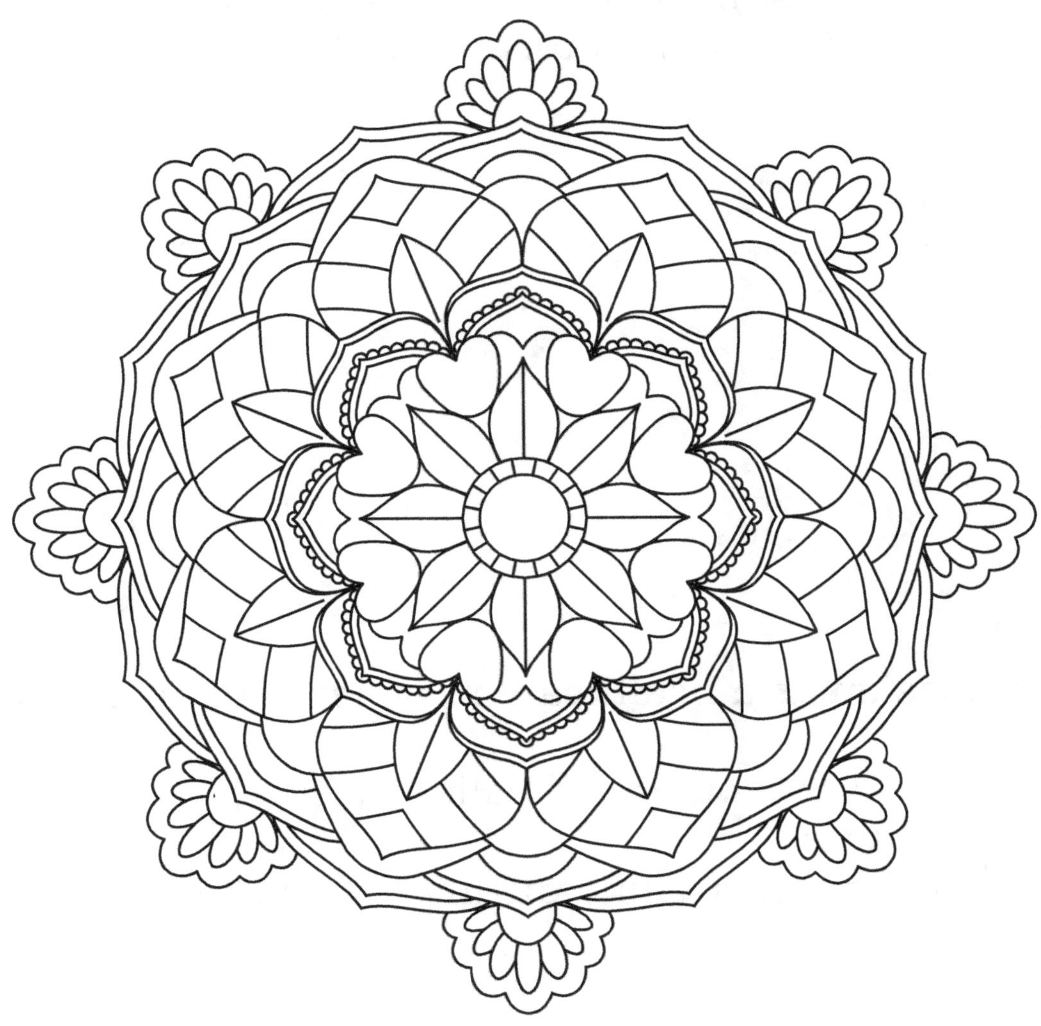

Affirmation: Positive energy nourishes me.

*"It is during our darkest moments
that we must focus to see the light."
— Aristotle Onasis*

Your mission as a healthcare provider is to help others.

You are a healing light.

Keep this in mind during difficult times.

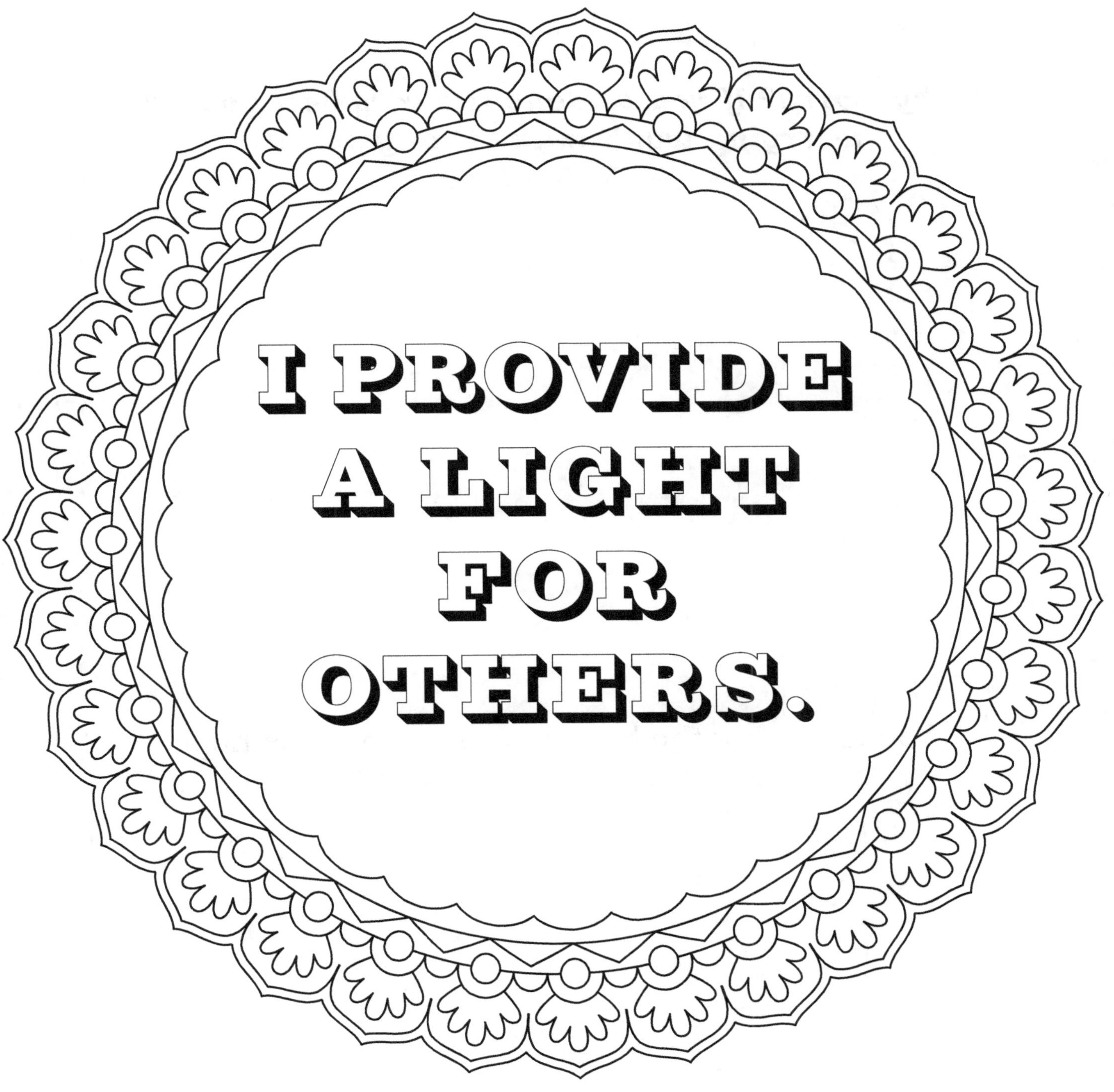

Affirmation: I provide a light for others.

*"Why worry? If you've done the very best you can,
worrying won't make it any better."*
— Walt Disney

You are doing the best you can to provide hope
and care to those in need.

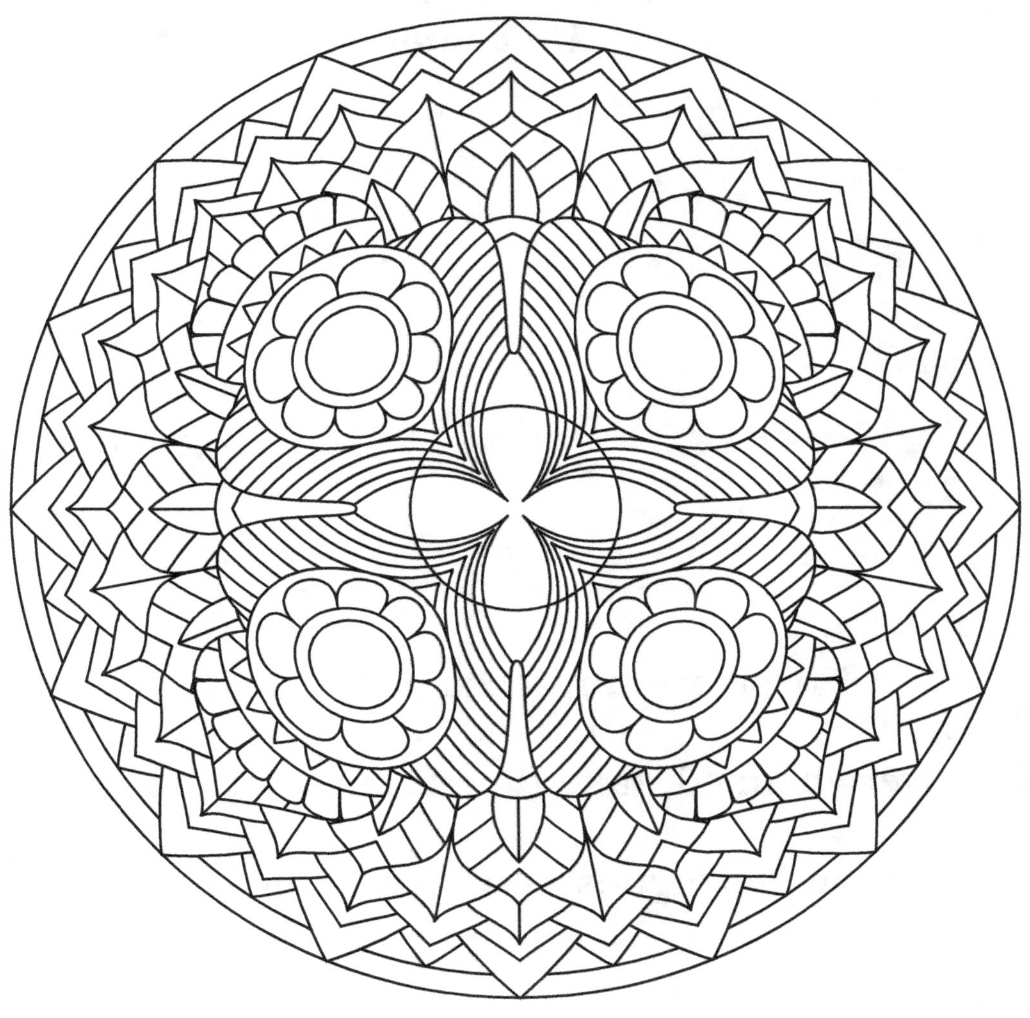

Affirmation: I do the best I can.

These are unprecedented times.

If you feel overwhelmed, take time to find your inner strength.

Lean on colleagues and friends for support.

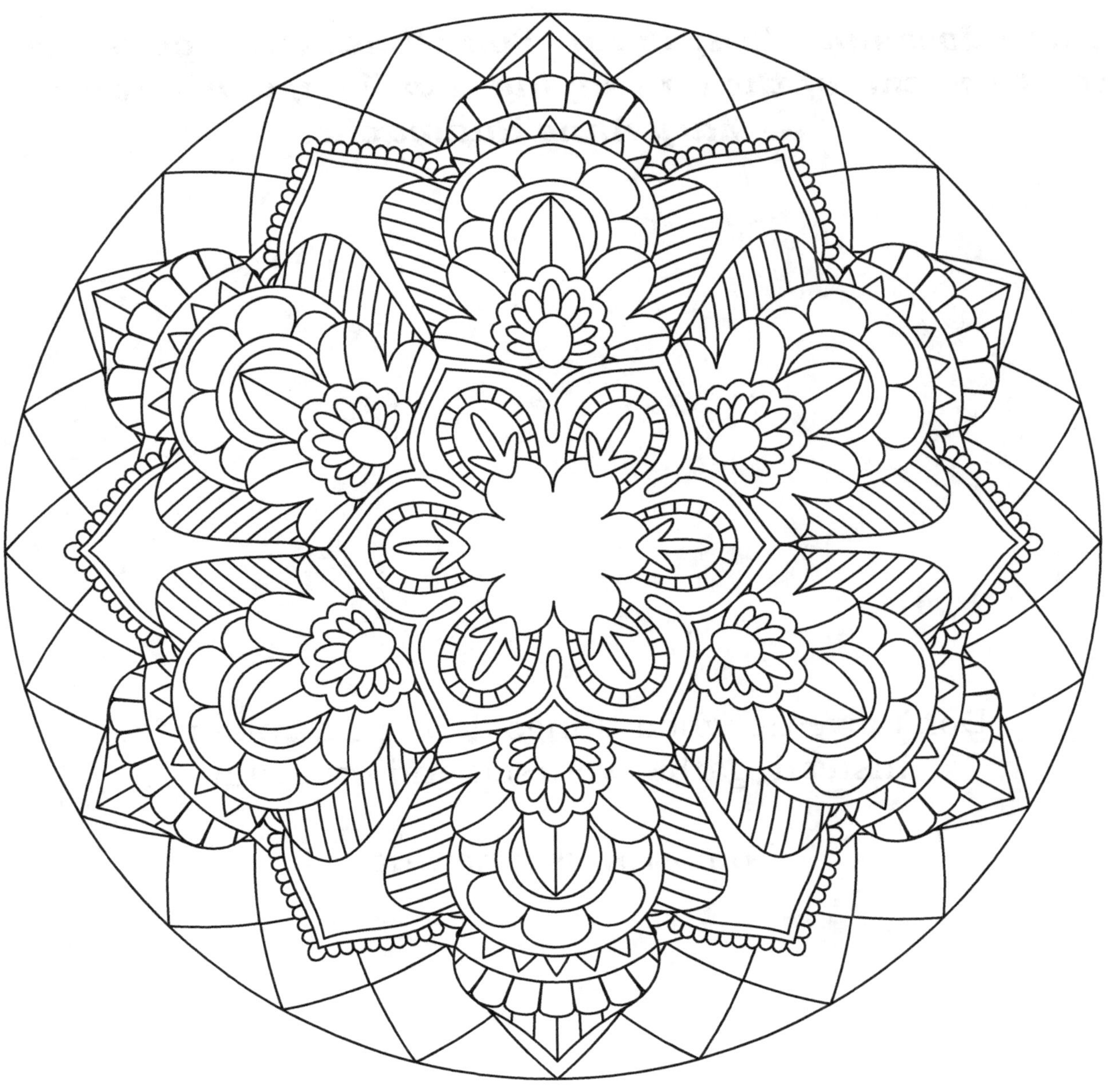

Affirmation: I am strong and determined.

"Courage does not always roar. Sometimes courage is the quiet voice at the end of the day saying, I will try again tomorrow."
— Mary Anne Radmacher

Don't give up when things don't go as planned.
Instead, gather yourself and try again.

Tomorrow is a new day.

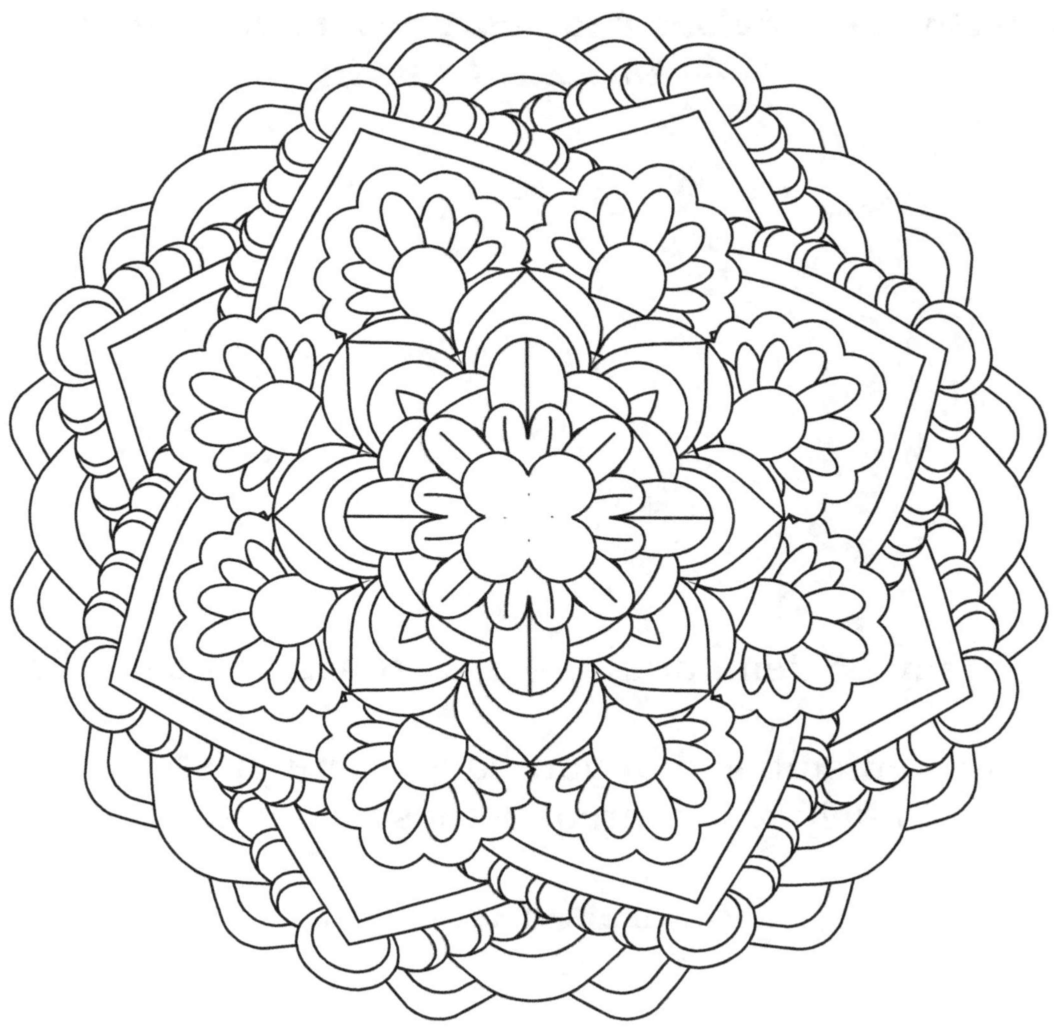

Affirmation: What I do today will create a brighter tomorrow.

*"It is only in our darkest hours that we may
discover the true strength of the brilliant
light within ourselves that can never, ever, be dimmed.
— Doe Zantamata*

Your work may be demanding, and at times you could lose hope.

But remember that you have an inner strength
to help you overcome these challenges.

You are a bright light.

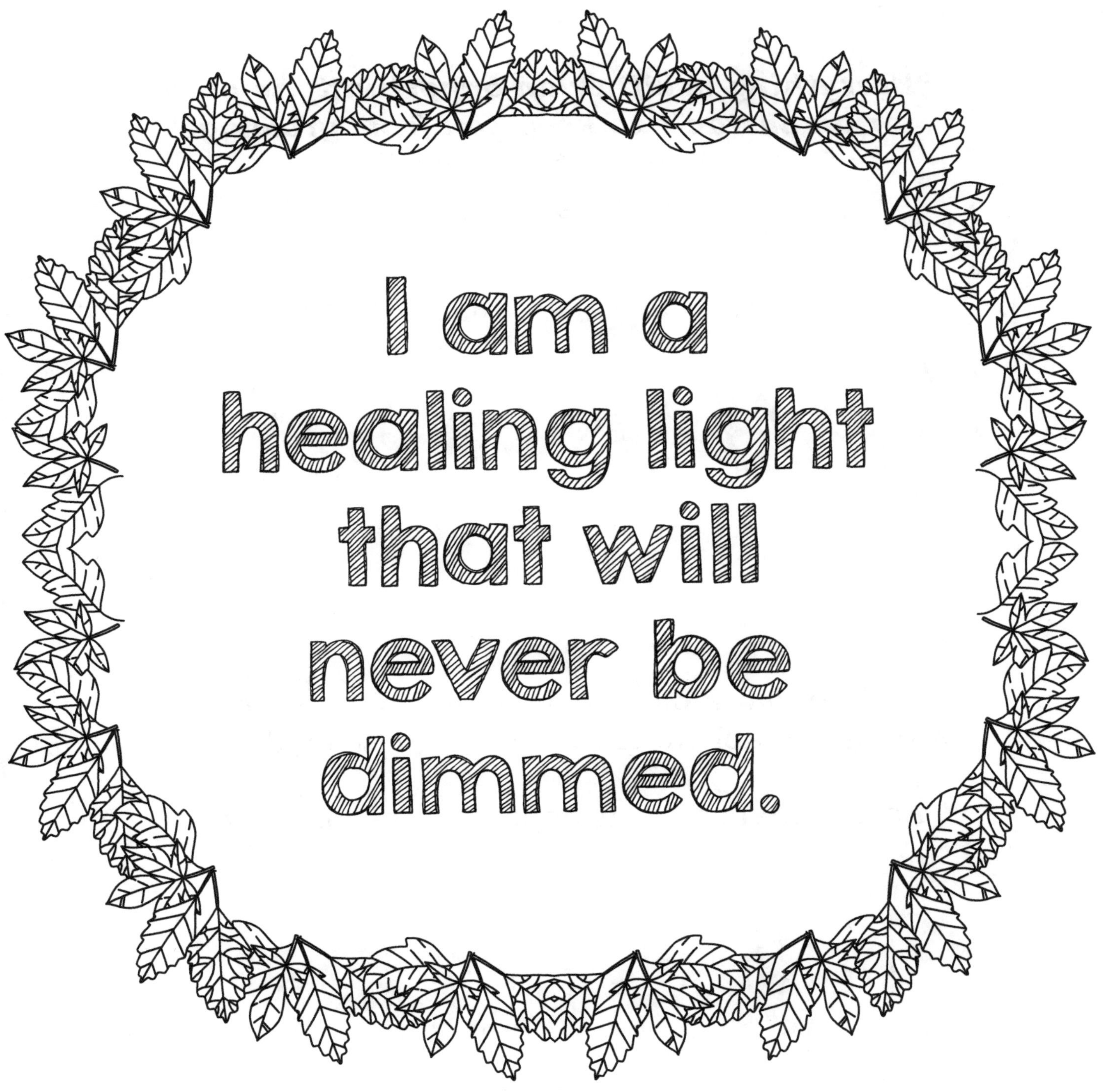

Affirmation: I am a healing light that will never be dimmed.

*"Everything is either an opportunity to grow
or an obstacle to keep you from growing.
You get to choose."*
— Wayne Dyer

Your work may be difficult, but you are
strong and able to grow beyond these challenges.

Accept challenges as opportunities for growth.

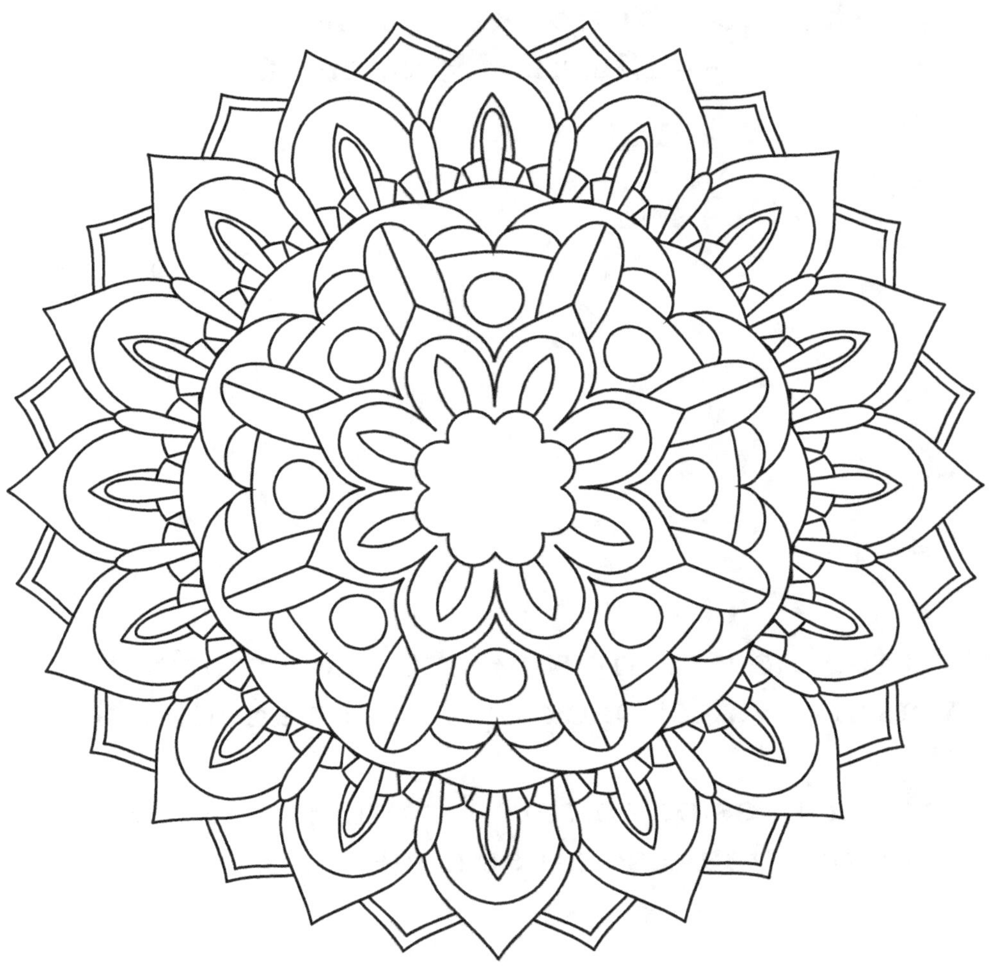

Affirmation: I look for ways to grow in
whatever comes my way.

"You gain strength, courage, and confidence by every experi-ence in which you really stop to look fear in the face. You are able to say to yourself, I lived through this horror. I can take the next thing that comes along."
— Eleanor Roosevelt

No matter how many times you get knocked down,
you always get back up to fight another day.

Your passion to care for others fuels you
and makes you stronger each day.

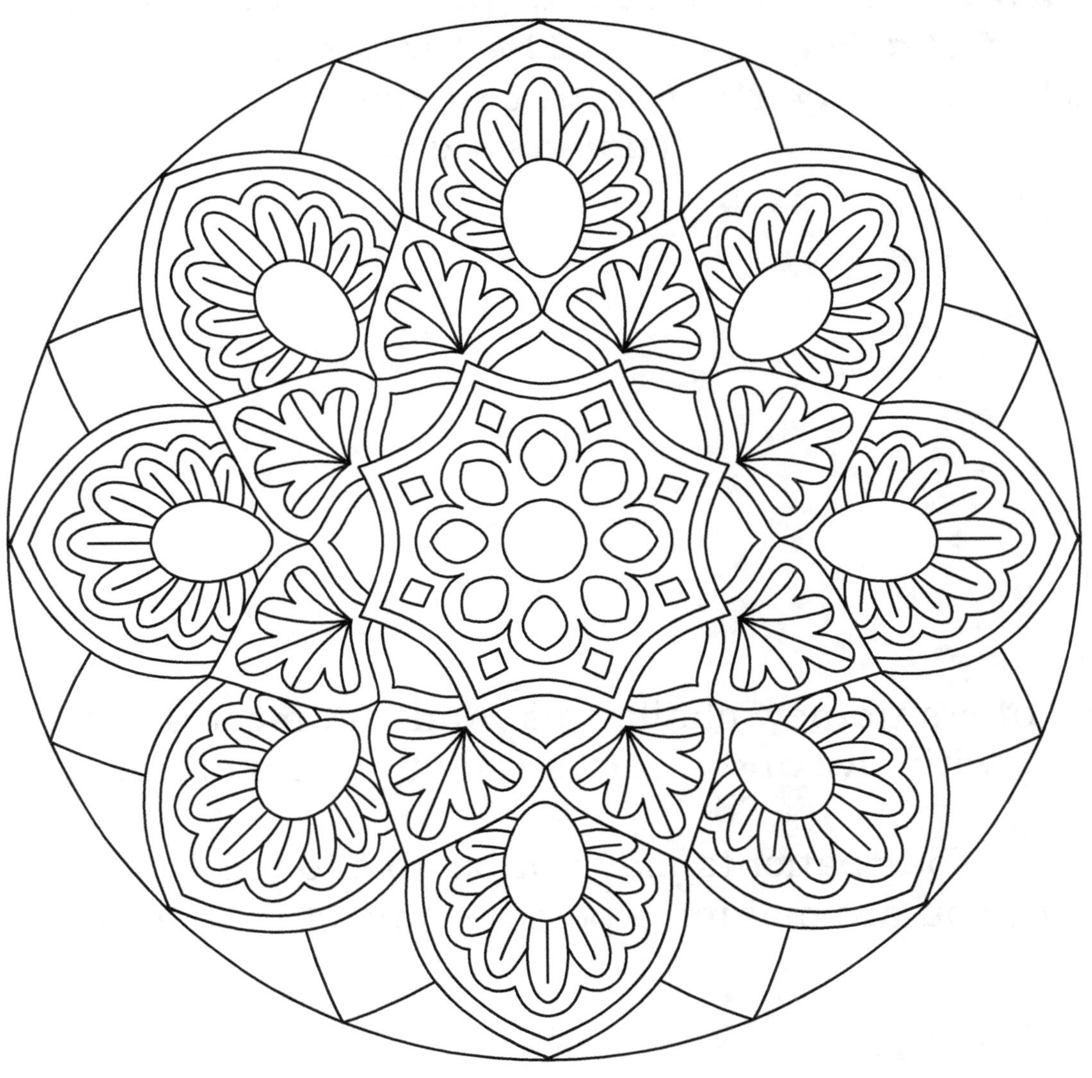

Affirmation: I will continue the fight.

*"You do not need to know precisely what
is happening, or exactly where it is all going.
What you need is to recognize the possibilities
and challenges offered by the present moment,
and to embrace them with courage, faith and hope."*
— Thomas Merton

Each day offers up new challenges. And you meet those challenges
with love and a commitment to help others.

Your patients may not be able to tell you,
but you are making a positive impact in their lives.

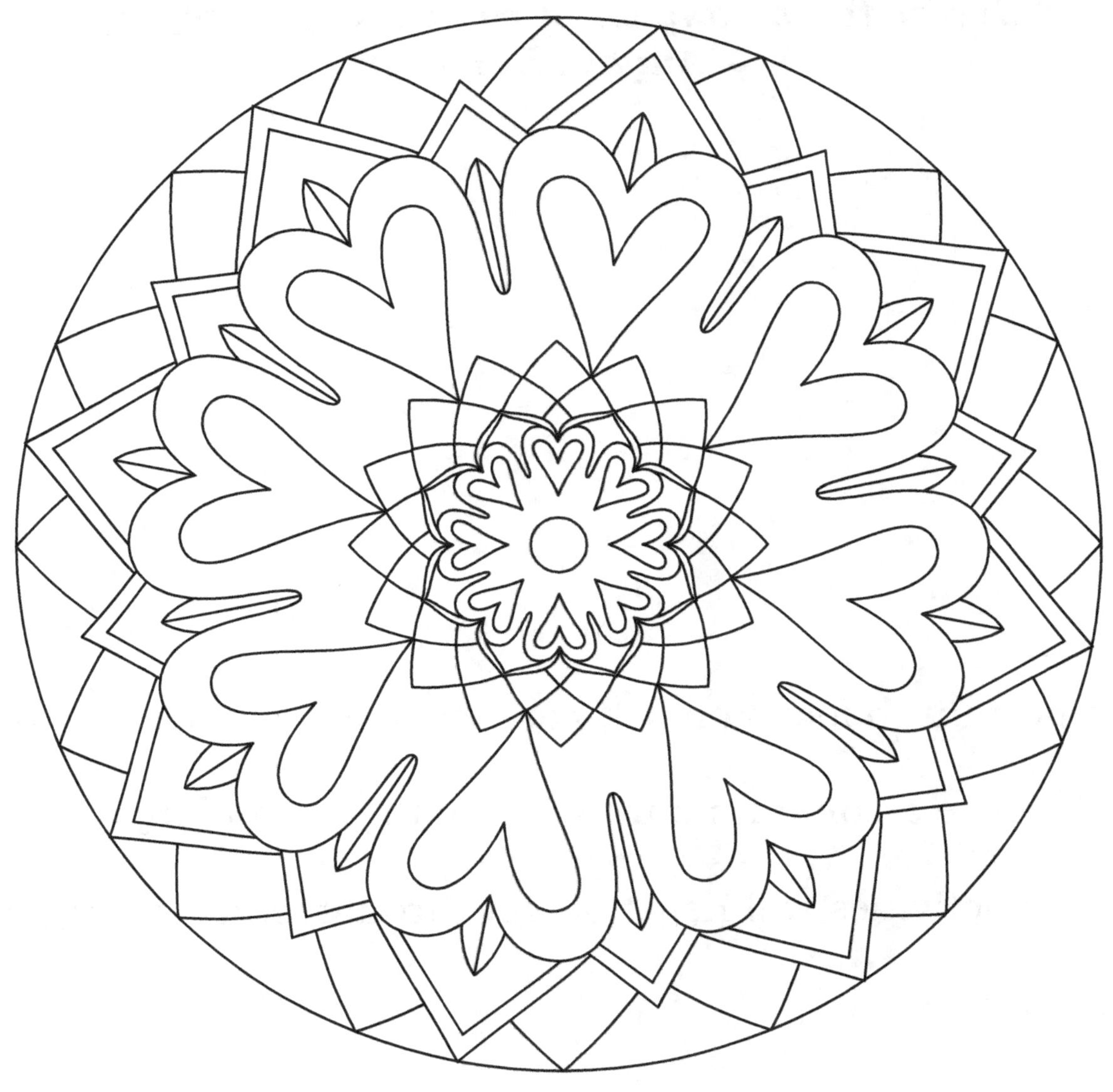

Affirmation: I am present for others in their time of greatest need.

"Better to be busy than to be busy worrying."
— Angela Lansbury

It's important to focus on self-care even as you care for others.

Make a commitment to do the things you enjoy.

Self-care activities will help you get through challenging times.

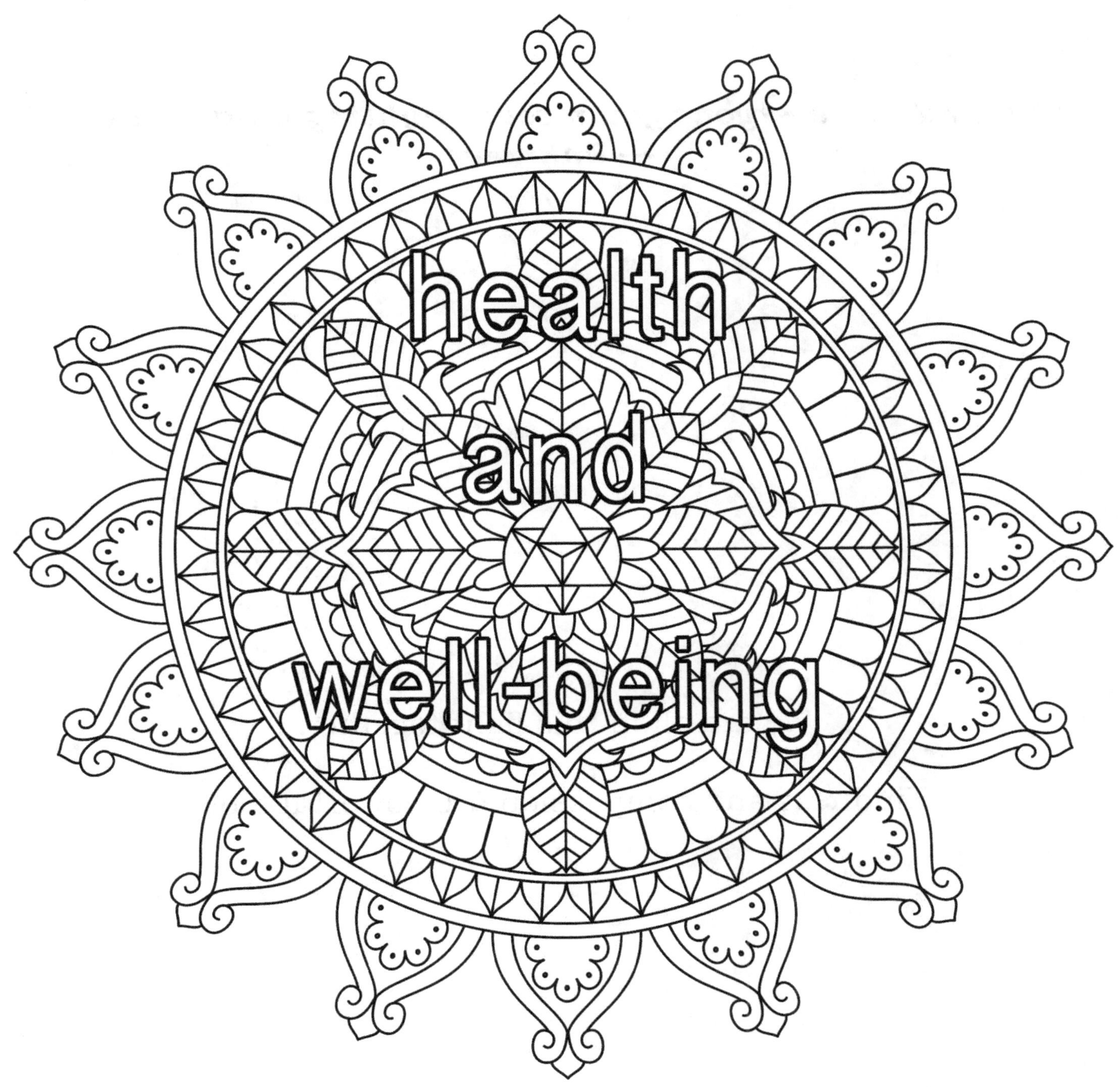

Affirmation: I will focus on activities that promote
my health and well-being.

"Be kind, for everyone you meet is fighting a hard battle."
— Unknown

We are all in this fight together.

Kindness and compassion are powerful tools.

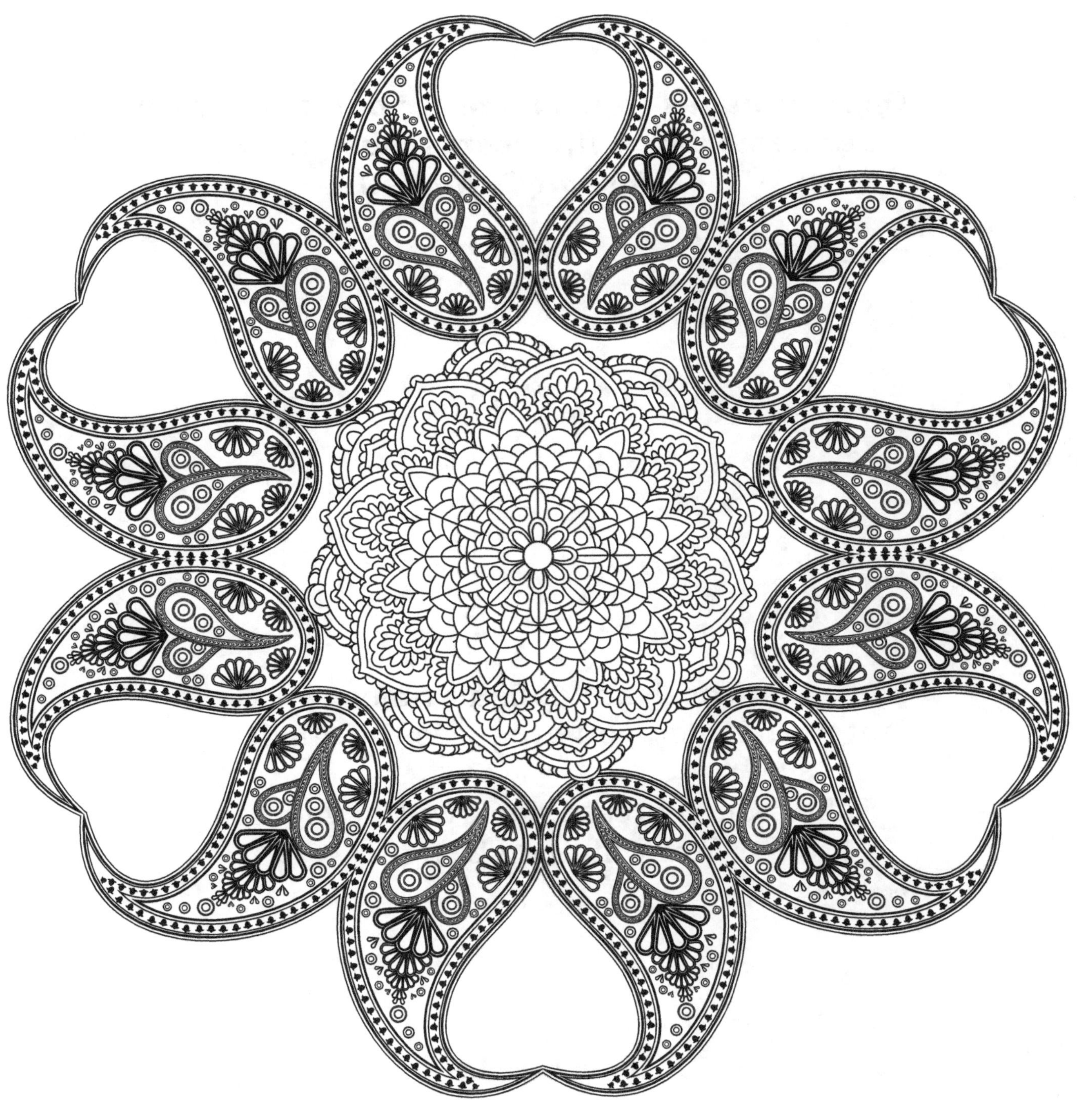

Affirmation: I focus on kindness and compassion.

"Opportunities to find deeper powers within ourselves come when life seems most challenging."
— Joseph Campbell

These are difficult times,
but as a healer, you are up to the challenge.

Take a deep breath, look within yourself.
You will find strength.

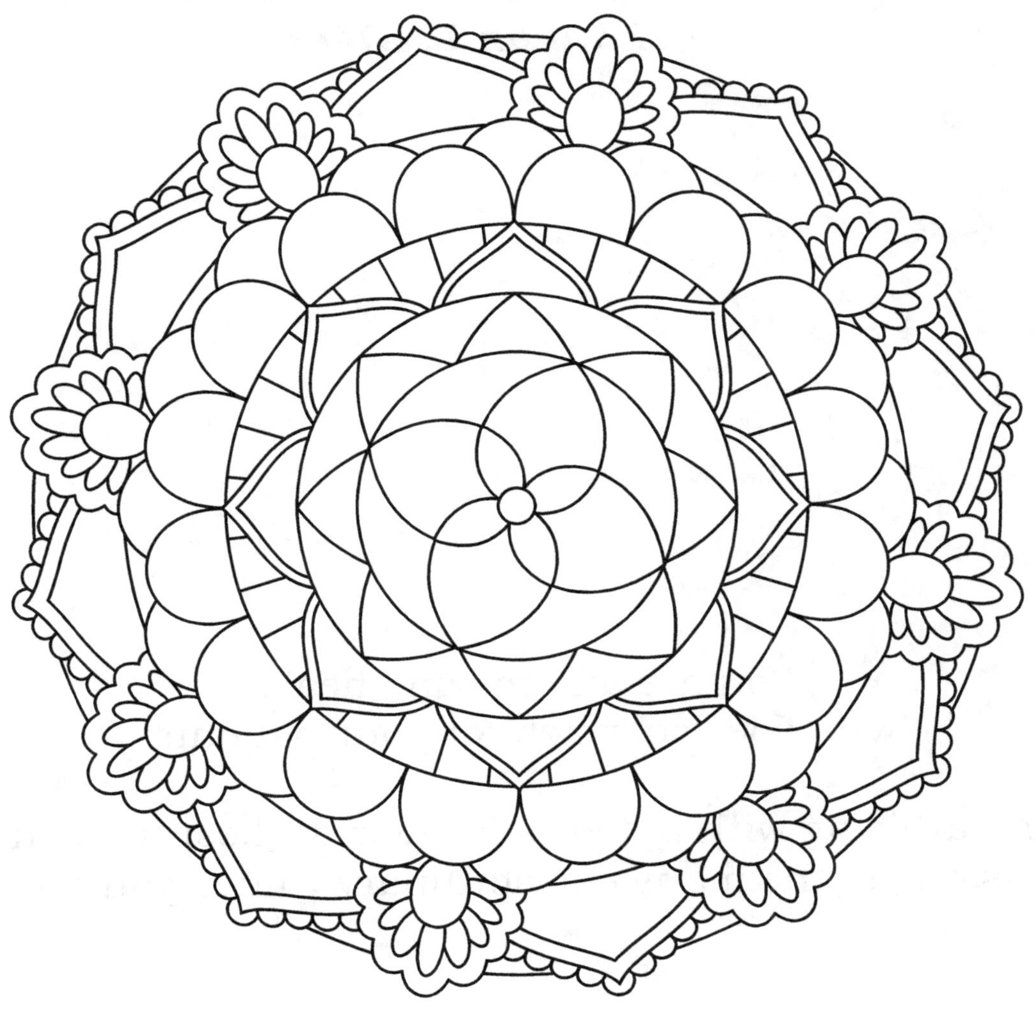

Affirmation: I find strength deep within myself.

*"One of the most important things we can do
on this earlth is to let people know they are not alone."*
— Shannon L. Alder

You are an amazing healer
who does so much for your patients.

Empathizing with patients in their darkest moments
is one of the many extraordinary things you do.

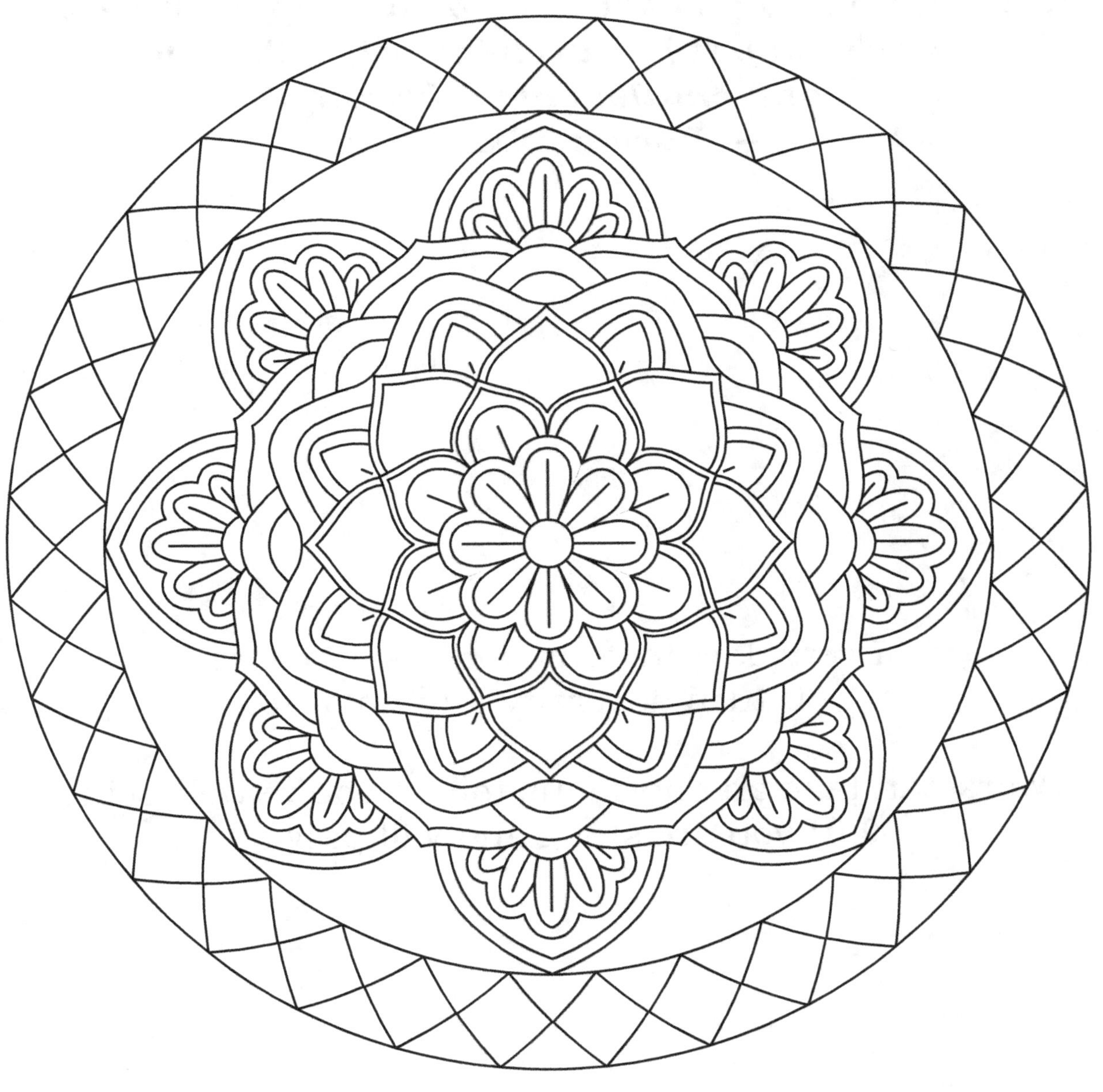

Affirmation: I let others know I am here for them.

Every day, in your work as a healer,
you turn adversity into an asset.

Work can take an enormous toll on you're well-being,
but you are stong and will prevail.

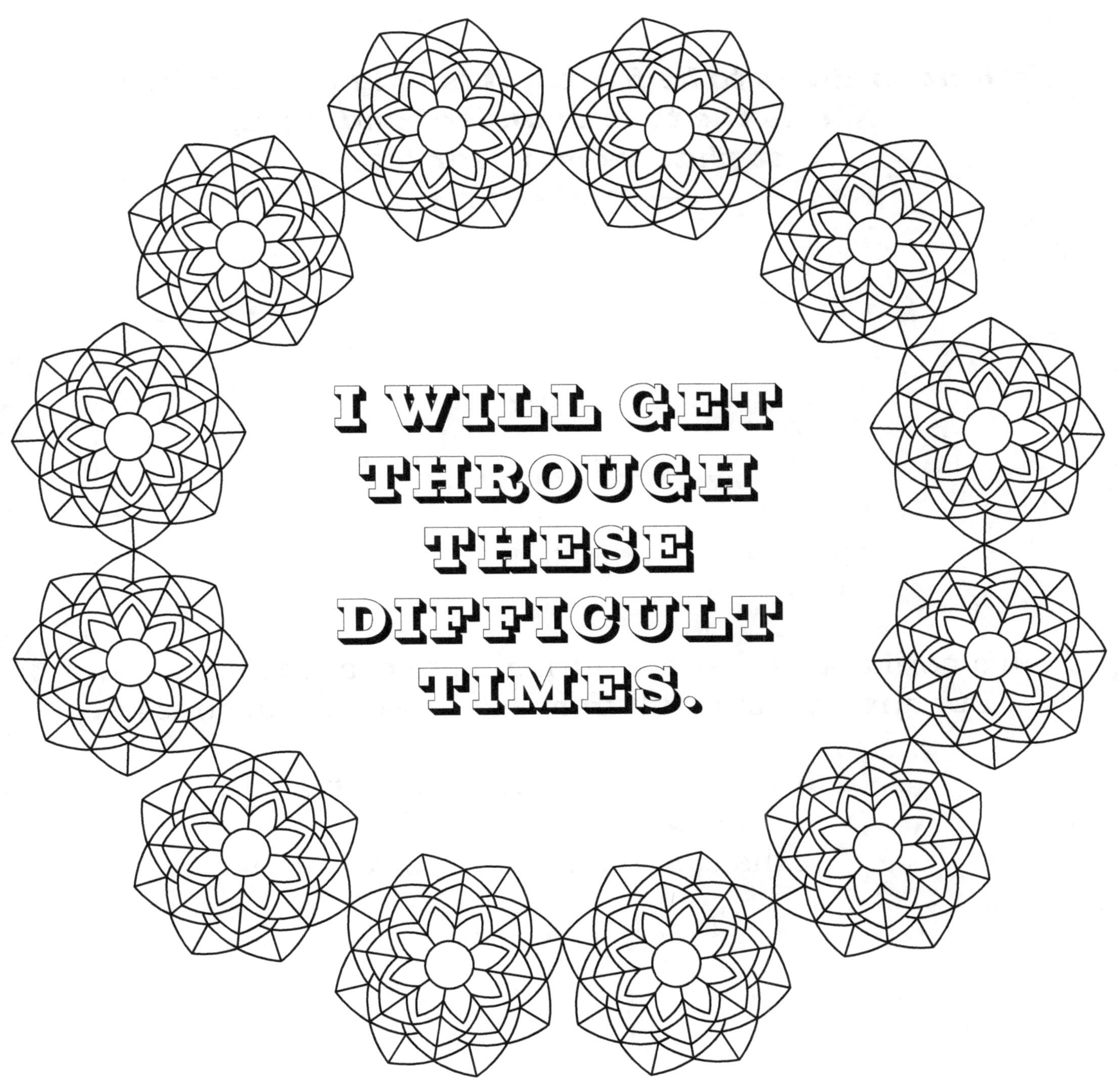

Affirmation: I am strong.

"Nothing in life is to be feared, it is only to be understood.
Now is the time to understand more,
so that we may fear less."
— Marie Curie

It's normal to feel stress during these challenging times.
But anxiety can result from excess worry and stress.

If you are experiencing anxiety,
draw in a deep breath,
exhale, and release the stress.

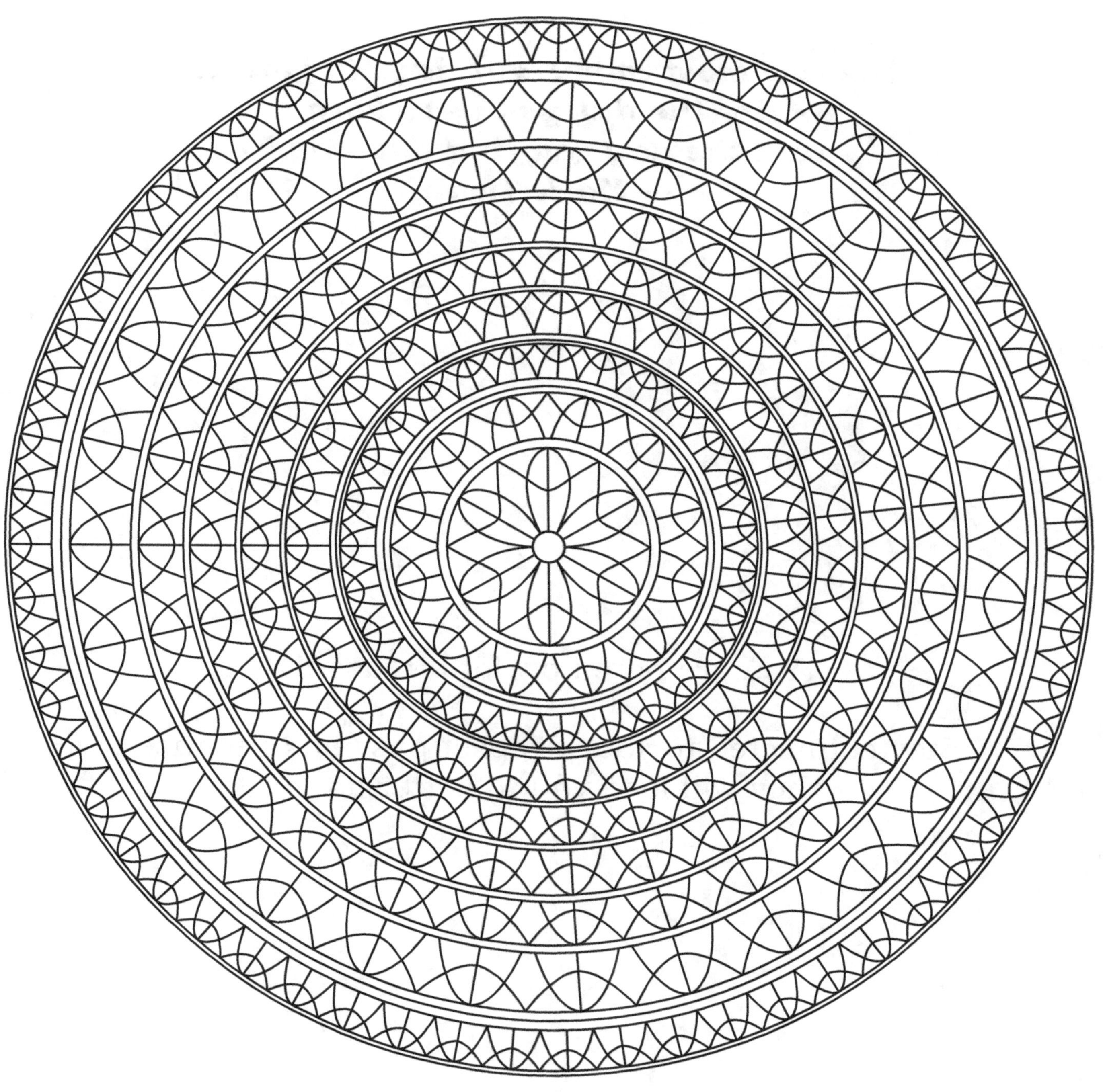

Affirmation: I will release fear and worry.

*"The two most important days in your life
are the day you were born
and the day you find out why."*
— Mark Twain

You are here now for a reason.

Stay connected to your deepest passions because
they will lead you to better days.

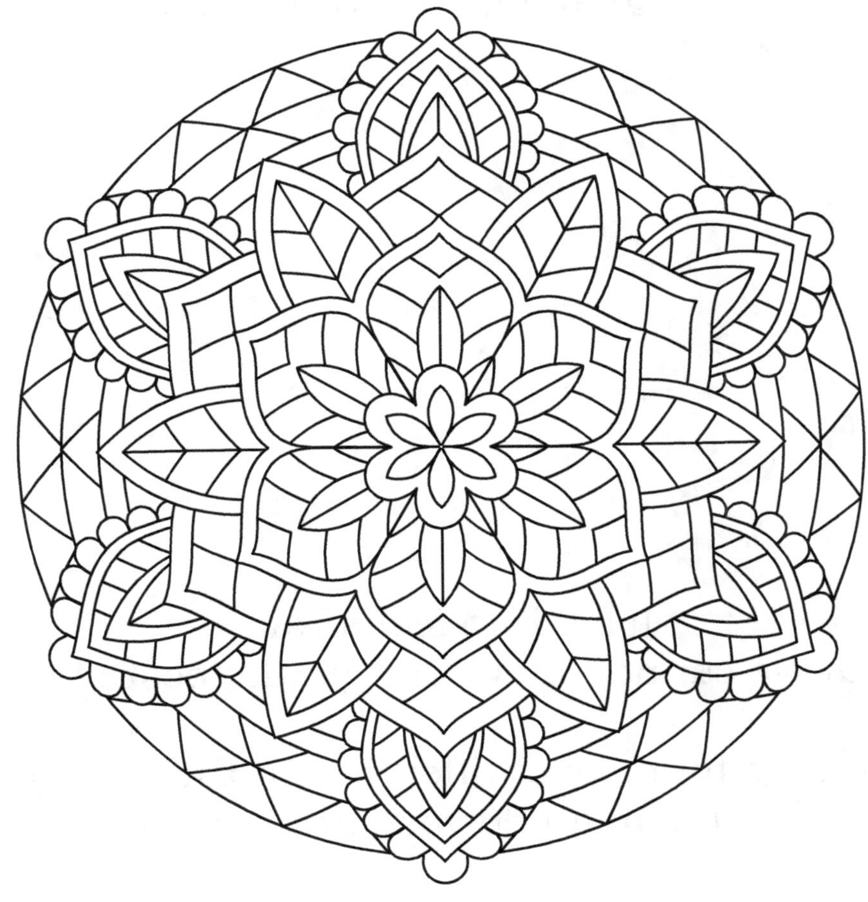

Affirmation: My dedication to help others brings meaning to my life.

*"Courage is not the absence of fear,
but rather the assessment that something else
is more important than fear."*
— Franklin D. Roosevelt

It's OK to feel afraid,
but we cannot allow fear get the best of us.

Your courage to make a difference in the lives of others
will help guide you through fear.

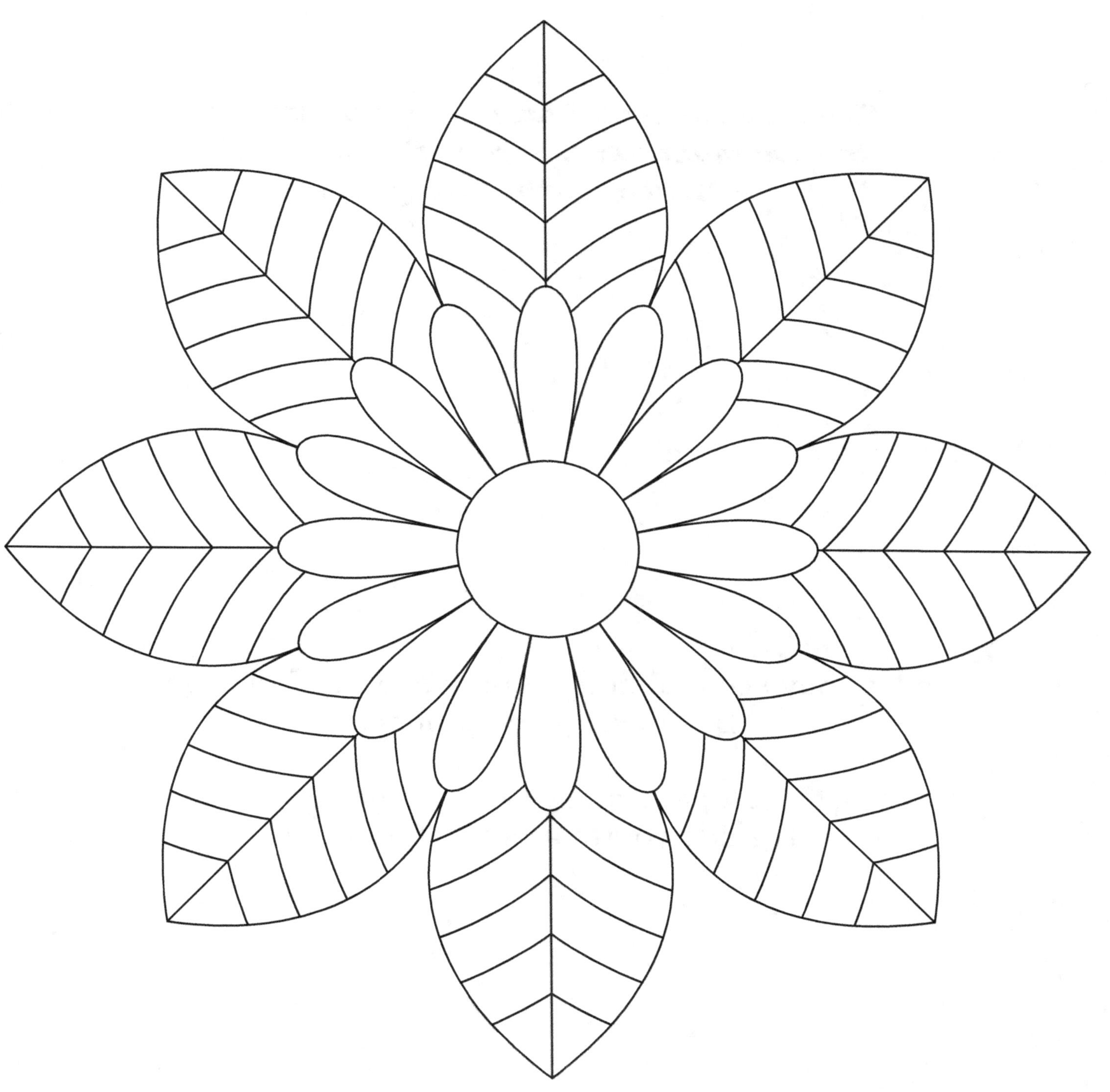

Affirmation: Courage will carry me forward.

***"We must accept finite disappointment,
but we must never lose infinite hope."
— Martin Luther King, Jr.***

Today may seem difficult. And it's OK to feel down.
But never give up hope.

Hope, along with courage,
will guide you to a better tomorrow.

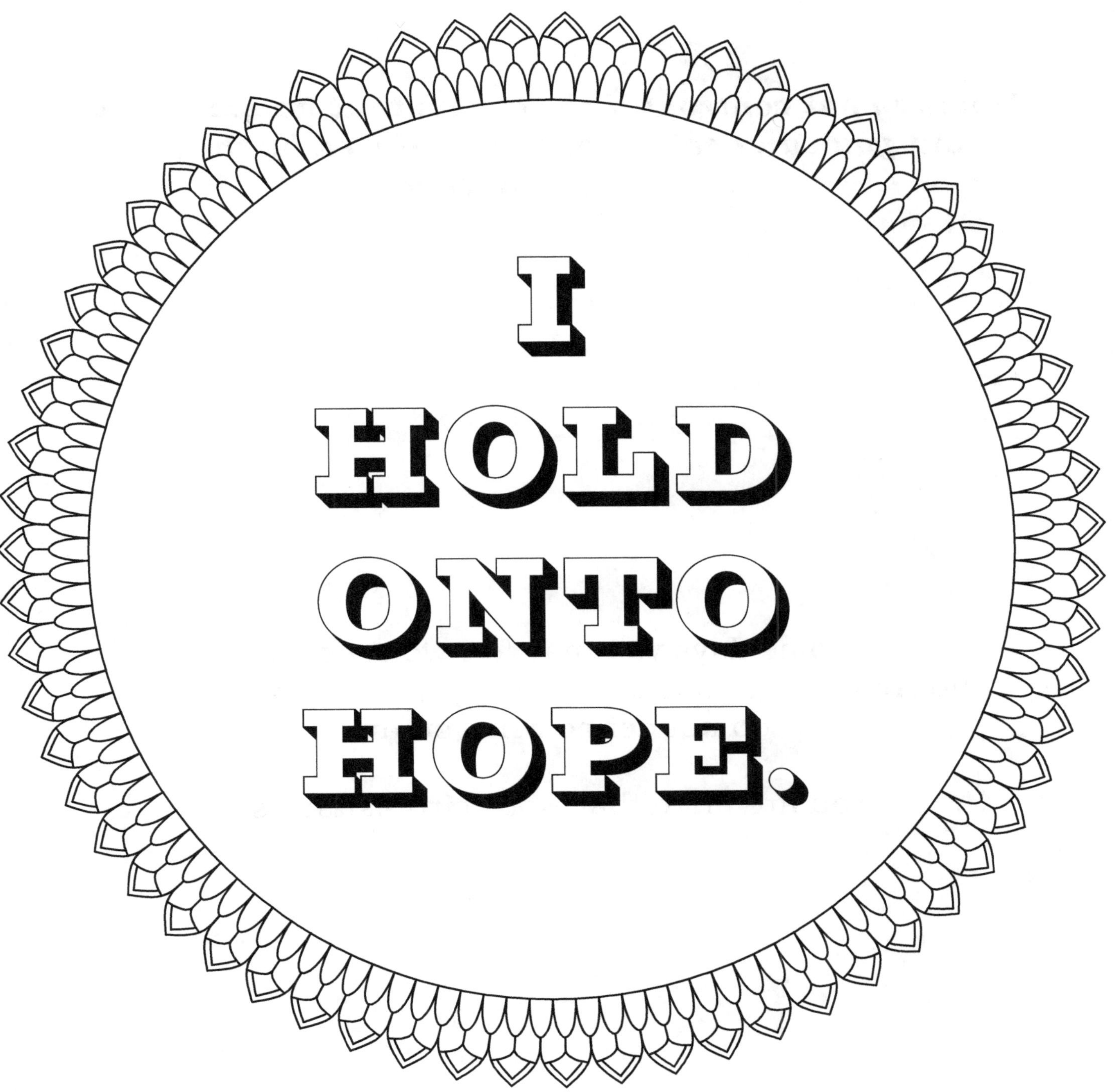

Affirmation: I hold onto hope.

*"You may not control all the events that happen to you,
but you can decide not to be reduced by them."*
— Maya Angelou

Some days you may feel worn down,
but remember that the events going on around you
do not define who you are.

You are more than your cirumstances.

Don't give up.

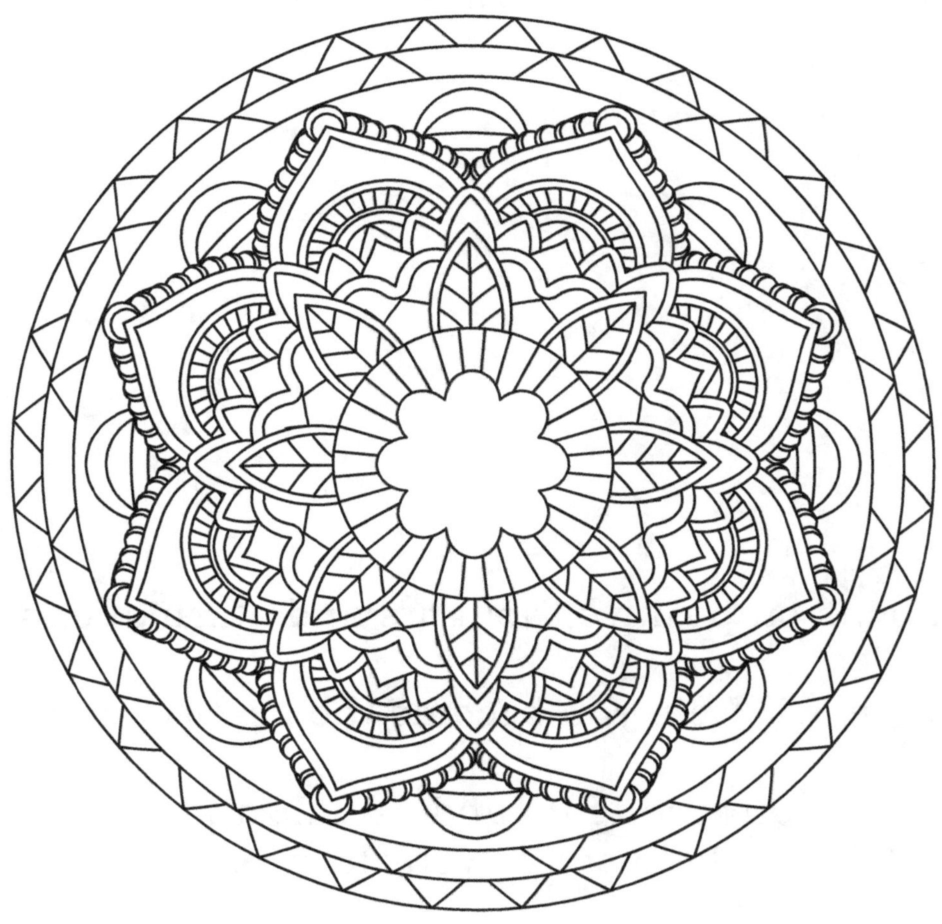

Affirmation: I decide what defines me.

"A man is but the product of his thoughts.
What he thinks, he becomes."
— Mahatma Gandhi

Focus on positive thoughts and affirmations.

This technique will help you become the best version of yourself.

Your thoughts and visualizations
help create your future.

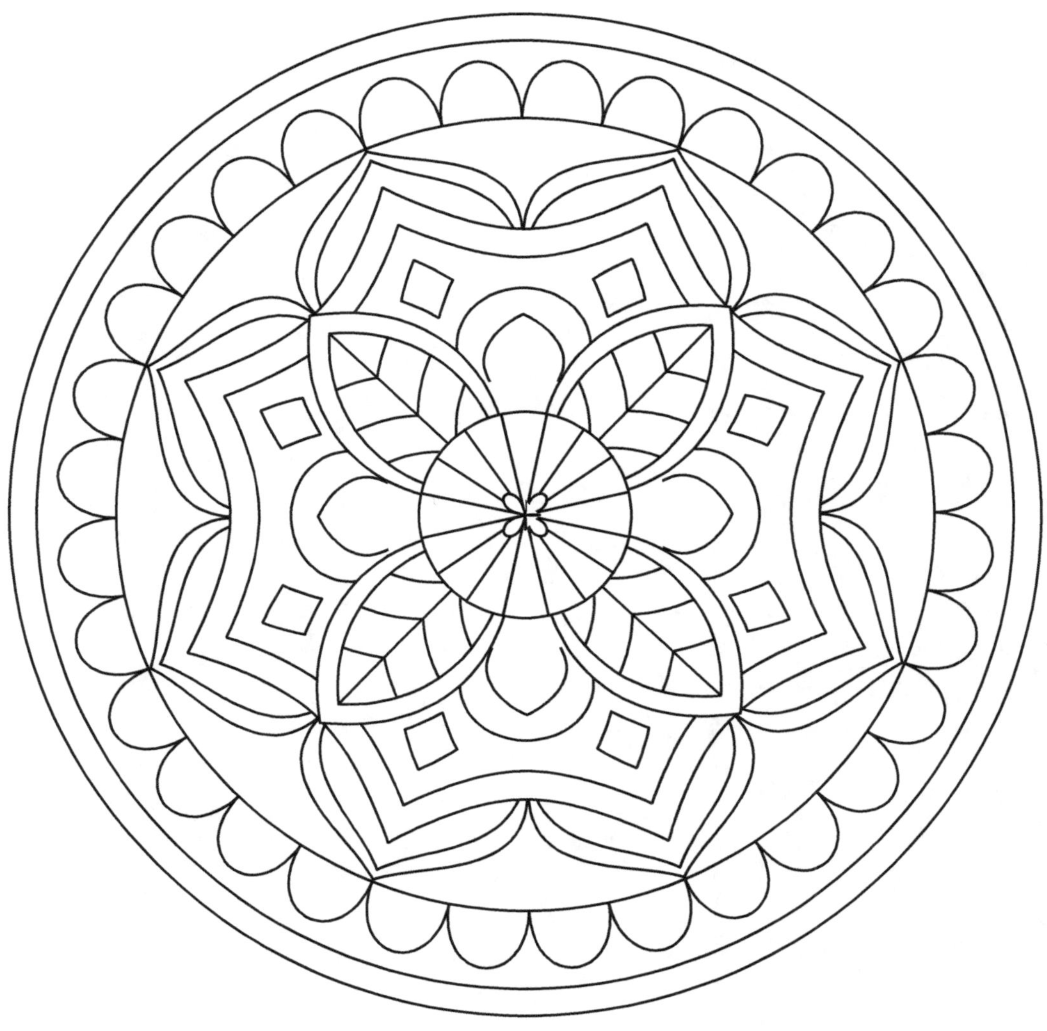

Affirmation: I visualize a positive future.